HEAL

DISCOVER YOUR UNLIMITED POTENTIAL AND AWAKEN THE POWERFUL HEALER WITHIN

KELLY NOONAN GORES

ATRIA PAPERBACK
New York London Toronto Sydney New Delhi

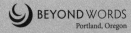
BEYOND WORDS
Portland, Oregon

ATRIA PAPERBACK
An Imprint of Simon & Schuster, Inc.
1230 Avenue of the Americas
New York, NY 10020

BEYOND WORDS
1750 S.W. Skyline Blvd., Suite 20
Portland, Oregon 97221-2543
503-531-8700 / 503-531-8773 fax
www.beyondword.com

Managing Editor: Lindsay S. Easterbrooks-Brown
Editors: Linda M. Meyer, Emily Han, Michele Cohn
Proofreader: Ashley Van Winkle
Design: Devon Smith

Simon + Schuster: Celebrating 100 Years of Publishing in 2024

First Beyond Words/Atria Books paperback edition January 2024

ATRIA PAPERBACK and colophon are trademarks of Simon & Schuster, Inc.

BEYOND WORDS PUBLISHING and colophon are registered trademarks of Beyond Words Publishing. Beyond Words is an imprint of Simon & Schuster, Inc.

For information about special discounts for bulk purchases, please contact Simon & Schuster Special Sales at 1-866-506-1949 or business@simonandschuster.com.

The Simon & Schuster Bureau can bring authors to your live event. For more information or to book an event, contact Simon & Schuster Speakers Bureau at 1-866-248-3049 or visit our website at www.simonspeakers.com.

Manufactured in the United States of America

10 9 8 7 6 5 4 3 2 1

Library of Congress Cataloging-in-Publication Data

Names: Noonan Gores, Kelly, author.
Title: Heal : discover your unlimited potential and awaken the powerful
  healer within / Kelly Noonan Gores.
Description: First Beyond Words hardback edition. | New York : Atria Hardcover;
  Hillsboro, Oregon : Beyond Words, 2019. | Includes bibliographical references.
Identifiers: LCCN 2019008862 (print) | LCCN 2019020606 (ebook) |
  ISBN 9781582707273 (eBook) | ISBN 9781582707129 (hardcover)
Subjects: LCSH: Healing. | Health. | Healing—Psychological aspects. | Medicine.
Classification: LCC RA776.5 (ebook) | LCC RA776.5 .N66 2019 (print) |
  DDC 613—dc23
LC record available at https://lccn.loc.gov/2019008862

ISBN: 978-1-58270-922-2 (paperback)

The corporate mission of Beyond Words Publishing, Inc.: *Inspire to Integrity*

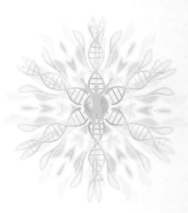

This book is dedicated to you, the reader,
wherever you find yourself on your healing journey.
May it help to awaken the powerful healer within
and support you on the road back to vibrant health.

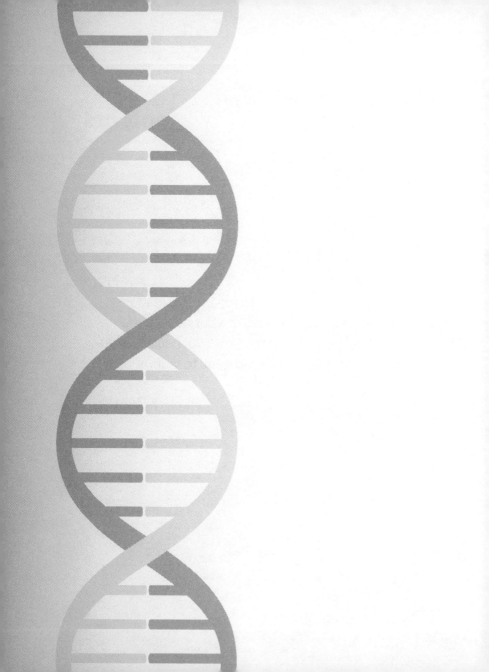

Contents

Foreword

What an amazing time to be alive. Since the turn of the millennium, more than at any other time in human history, information has become increasingly and more readily available. We are living in a brave new world. As a consequence of this great age of information, to remain ignorant is a choice.

With the advent of technology, we are being exponentially empowered in countless new ways—every day. Having information at our fingertips affords us the ability to make new, different, and better choices. No longer do we need a teacher or a formal education to access information that was once only in the hands of authorities, experts, and gatekeepers. By the same means, people all over the world are more motivated than ever to proactively research their own diagnosis and then make significant, corresponding lifestyle changes. Millions of people are now seeking alternative treatments for their health conditions (without consulting a doctor or blindly taking medication), and they are experiencing considerable results. Still others, without the aid of a priest, minister, or a rabbi, are taking the time to delve deeply into well-researched understandings about ancient religions, theology, and the nature of reality. Through these inquiries, they are having profound mystical experiences that positively alter them for the rest of their lives.

When you gain information, the understanding of new knowledge creates a greater sense of awareness about yourself and the world around you. It lifts you above the mundane, routine way in which you see reality. A new awareness about some "thing" creates a new level of consciousness, and when there is a change in consciousness, there is a change in energy. The outcome is that you are empowered and awakened by knowledge. Why? Because knowledge is, has always been, and will always be power.

Thus, when you learn about yourself, you empower yourself. In a sense, you reclaim your power by no longer believing you are a helpless victim—one who blindly accepts having no ability or authority to change one's life. Gaining knowledge can cause you to cease unconsciously giving your power away to (or relying on) someone or something to do things for you. This is why the age of information is making way for a new era of consciousness.

From a neuroscientific standpoint, learning is making new synaptic connections. Every time you learn something new, your brain assembles thousands of new circuits, which are reflected as patterns in your gray matter. The latest brain science research demonstrates that when you focus your attention for one hour on a concept or idea, the number of connections in your brain literally doubles. These new footprints of consciousness are the physical evidence that you learned through interacting with your environment. However, the same research shows that if you don't repeatedly think about what you've learned, or take the time to review the new information over and over again, those circuits will prune apart within hours or days. If learning is making new synaptic connections, then remembering is maintaining or sustaining those new connections.

With just a little concentration and repetition, intellectual information becomes embossed in your biology. This is how knowledge changes you. We don't see things the way they are, we see things the way *we* are. A different lens of how you perceive the world is inserted into your brain, and as a side effect you see new possibilities—possibilities you were unaware of prior to your interaction with knowledge. That's because your brain only "sees" equal to how it's wired, which implies that you can only see what you know.

While people do their best with what they know is available, if they don't know about something, we could say that it doesn't exist for them. In the same way, we could say that once they become aware or conscious of it, it comes into existence. In this manner, however, the acquisition of such knowledge is void of experience. When you can see a new potential reality or possibility, it's time to do something with that knowledge.

What all of this comes down to is that the more you know what you're doing and why, the *how* to do it gets easier. That's why this is a time in history when it's not enough to simply *know*—it's a time to *know how*.

As a seeker of truth, knowledge, wisdom, and information, your next job is to initiate that knowledge by applying, personalizing, or demonstrating what you philosophically and theoretically learned. This means you're going to have to make new and different choices that will require you to get your body involved. When you can align your behaviors with your intentions, your actions equal to your thoughts— get your mind and body working together—you are going to have a new experience.

Experience enriches the synaptic connections in your brain. When you embrace a novel experience, the new event adds to—and enhances—the intellectual circuitry in your brain. The moment those circuits further organize into new networks, the brain makes a corresponding chemical. We call this chemical a feeling or an emotion. The instant you feel more vitality, better health, wholeness, or joy from that novel event, you're teaching your body chemically to understand what your mind has understood intellectually. Now new information is making its way to your body, not just to your mind, and it's changing your state of being. In truth, you are conditioning your body to a new mind. And in that moment, mind and body are aligned to new information.

It's fair to say, then, that knowledge is for the mind, and experience is for the body. Now you are beginning to *embody the truth* of that philosophy. In doing so, you're rewriting your biological program and signaling new genes in new ways, because new information is coming from the environment. As we know from epigenetics, if the environment signals genes, and the end product of an experience in the environment is an emotion, you are literally signaling genes in new ways. And since all genes make proteins, and proteins are responsible for the structure and function of your body (the expression of proteins is the expression of life), you are literally changing your genetic destiny. This suggests that it's quite possible that your body can be healed in an instant.

Accordingly, if you can create an experience once, you should be able to do it again. When you keep making the same choices and reproducing the same experiences over and over again, eventually you will neurochemically condition your mind and body to begin to work as one. When you've done something so many times that the body knows how to do it as well as the mind, it becomes automatic, natural, and effortless. Simply said, now it has become a skill, a habit, or a way of life. Once you've achieved that level of competence, you no longer have to consciously think about performing that task. That's when you've truly changed your state of being, because the information is innate in you. You're beginning to *master that philosophy*. You have become that knowledge.

The outcome of your repeated efforts will not only change who you are, but it also should create even more possibilities in your life that are a reflection of your efforts. Why else would you do it? And what do I mean when I say *possibilities*? I'm talking about healing from diseases or imbalances of both the body and the mind. I'm talking about creating a better life for yourself by no longer making the same unconscious choices programmed from past traumas. When you eliminate those choices, behaviors, and experiences, and you live by new choices, behaviors, and experiences, the results can come in the form of new jobs, new relationships, new opportunities, and new life adventures.

This book and the *Heal* documentary are part of a new and different genre of journalism that comprises so much more than just a group of scientists, researchers, or healers espousing theories about how you can change your health. Because you can witness real people—just like you—experimenting with different modalities that might actually change their health, *Heal* is a practical and real study of healing. These stories of personal change and transformation are not Hollywood versions of glamorous triumph-against-all-odds stories. Instead, in order to make significant strides in their recovery, these are accounts of common people who have had to look deeply into themselves to see what it was they needed to continually change in their thoughts, feelings, and deeds. These accounts are real and relatable.

When I was first approached by Kelly Noonan Gores to be a part of the *Heal* documentary, I was overjoyed to know that someone was taking on a whole new level of investigation into what it takes to heal from chronic health conditions. I was relieved to know that her work provides evidence, which is the next level of information. Evidence is the most important voice.

Someone had to tell this story, and I am overjoyed that Kelly took it on with such sincerity, clarity, and open-mindedness. What it demonstrates is that it *is* possible that the mind can heal the body. In fact, my research team and I have conducted several experiments to show that most healings begin in the mind. We now know that there is never a time when your mind is not influencing your body, and there is never a moment when your body is not influencing your mind. This means that in order to change your body, you have to change your mind—and vice versa. Consider the idea that in order to begin your healing journey, you must first become aware of what you're thinking about, and then literally change your thoughts and feelings.

The long-term effects of stress hormones can push genetic buttons and create disease. Stress is when brain and body are knocked out of homeostasis, and it's the body's stress response that innately returns the body to balance. To live in stress is to live in a constant state of emergency and survival. Living in emergency mode for extended periods of time depletes the body's natural healing resources. All organisms in nature can tolerate short-term stress, but when we are under constant stress, the stress response is turned on and we can't turn it off. Now we're headed for disease. Simply said, if we are using all of our body's vital energy for some threat—*real* or *imagined*—in our outer world, there is no energy in our inner world for growth and repair.

Because of the size of the human forebrain and neocortex, we have the ability to make thought more real than anything else. This suggests that the stress response can be triggered simply by thinking about our problems or by anticipating future worst-case scenarios. Ponder that for a moment. Your thoughts can literally make you sick. This is a solid example of the mind-body connection. It begs the question, *If your thoughts can make you sick, is it possible that your thoughts can make you well?*

You will learn in this book that the answer is *yes.*

It has been my experience in working with chronic health conditions for more than thirty years that if there are three types of stressors (physical, chemical, and emotional) that create imbalance in the body, then there are three ways to create balance in the body—physically, chemically, and emotionally. Yoga, acupuncture, exercise, chiropractic, and massage can all counteract physical stress to create physical balance in the body. Making better food choices, reducing calories, and taking vitamins, herbs, or medications can combine to create better chemical balance. The summation of learning how to calm your mind and become more aware of your thoughts and feelings generates emotional balance. And meditation, energy psychology, eye movement desensitization and reprocessing (EMDR), emotional freedom technique (EFT), or psychotherapy all bring us back to neuro-emotional balance.

It has been my understanding that if you can recalibrate two out of three of these systems, bring them back into balance, in time the third system typically comes around. For example, if someone becomes more physically and chemically balanced, they will be more emotionally balanced. If they can become more chemically and emotionally balanced, more than likely they will become more physically balanced. By the same token, if they can become more physically and emotionally balanced, they will be more chemically balanced.

That's what this book is about. It's a guide to helping you find balance and health. As you will learn, Western medicine serves as a fabulous resource for acute health conditions. If you break your arm or develop appendicitis, your first choice should be to seek medical care. However, actually healing from chronic health conditions requires a lifestyle change. Simply taking a drug or a handful of drugs to mitigate your health condition is not healing. To truly heal, you must change the way you think, act, and feel. The totality of thinking, acting, and feeling makes up your personality, and your personality creates your personal reality. Change your personality and you change your personal reality.

What I have found in studying thousands of cases over the last twenty years, is that to heal is to, in a sense, become someone else.

Kelly and I share the belief that just as an infection can spread among a community and create disease, health and wellness can become as infectious as any disease. It's no small task to demystify how we heal, not to mention articulate it in a way accessible to the masses. Kelly has done a brilliant job in showing you what is possible.

Read this wonderful book with an open mind, and then make time to apply its principles in some way on a daily basis. After all, it was written to change your life.

Thank you, Kelly.

—Dr. Joe Dispenza
New York Times bestselling author of
You Are the Placebo: Making Your Mind Matter

Introduction

It was about ten years ago when I first considered filming a documentary about the incredible ability our bodies have for healing, and the powerful effect our minds have on our health and life. The initial seed was planted after reading Bruce Lipton's book *The Biology of Belief: Unleashing the Power of Consciousness, Matter, and Miracles.* I remember thinking: *We aren't victims of our genes? Everybody needs to know this!* Attending Dr. Michael B. Beckwith's services at Agape International Spiritual Center proved to be the rich soil from which that seed would grow. Not only did his teachings affirm the power of our thoughts and beliefs to influence our experience and our physical health, Dr. Beckwith's words inspired me to follow my heart and realize my vision of the documentary. He taught me that when you are pulled by a vision, it is a sign that you are aligned with your soul's purpose.

I started noticing how energized and passionate I became when discussing our minds in relation to our human potential to heal, motivating me to read, learn, and explore as much as I could on the topic. And then about three years ago, the final catalyst that set the film in motion was Anita Moorjani's book *Dying to Be Me: My Journey from Cancer, to Near Death, to True Healing*. The rush of inspiration I felt after reading her remarkable story gave me an inner confidence that I *had* to do this. *If Anita's physical body could heal from such a terrible diagnosis, then anyone's can!* In other words, divine timing had arrived; I finally felt ready to take the leap into the unknown and film a documentary with all my favorite teachers on the subject.

As it turned out, Dr. Beckwith's sermons didn't disappoint. The minute I listened to that pull and vision in my heart, the universe did indeed conspire to make it all happen. I would describe the process of making the film as a constant *flow* state. It wasn't without challenges and obstacles, but I felt an energy behind me that was beyond my own. That energy allowed me to surrender and trust that this documentary needed to be made, and I was just the messenger.

Upon release, the film was an immediate success. The positive response it received made me realize just how deeply it resonated with people, encouraging me to draw upon this momentum and create a book version to offer further support. I had always loved writing and I am an avid reader—the power of self-help books prompted my *Heal* journey—so this was the natural next step. A book would provide not only a tangible takeaway tool, allowing readers to easily revisit our *Heal* experts' powerful statements made in the film, but also an opportunity to delve into greater detail and depth than the film allowed.

Many have asked me if I was inspired to make the film *Heal* because I lost someone close to me to a devastating illness, or because I myself endured a difficult health challenge. The answer to both is, thankfully, no. But a few of my own (less dire) health issues helped spark an early interest in ancient and natural healing methods.

One such experience happened when I was a junior in high school. I came home from a camping trip at age sixteen and proceeded to get very sick with flu-like symptoms for a week. After recovering, my lymph nodes on my neck remained swollen for months. My doctor tested me for mononucleosis and Epstein-Barr virus, both of which came back negative. He gave me antibiotics to try to knock out the lingering infection—to no avail. When my golf ball–sized lymph nodes still protruded from my neck after ten months (not a good look for a gal in high school!), my doctor decided to do a lymph node biopsy. I went under general anesthesia and the surgeon made an inch-long incision on the left side of my neck. The biopsy came back normal and benign.

Some weeks later, I went with my mother to her chiropractic appointment after school. The chiropractor felt my glands and suggested I try drinking a one-to-two-ounce shot of apple cider vinegar each day for a week. My mom found a blueberry-flavored vinegar that was palatable, and I followed his instructions. Sure enough, eight days later my glands returned to their normal, healthy size. After visits to multiple doctors, a surgery, and three unsuccessful courses of antibiotics, I discovered my remedy in a bottle of vinegar bought at a health food store. This experience taught me that conventional doctors might not always know best. I began to awaken to a new sense of trust and love for alternative, natural modalities.

That growing curiosity about how the body works and how healers could promote successful remedies using nonconventional treatments has stayed with me. Throughout my journey, I've noted many areas where science and spirituality overlap, and it is fascinating to me that ancient healing modalities such as acupuncture, energy medicine, herbs, and meditation have been used successfully for thousands of years, yet still aren't widely recognized in conventional medicine. It is this wonderment and inquisitiveness that I take with me in my investigations into ancient and new frontiers of healing and wellness.

I am not a doctor of medicine. I am not a scientist. I am solely an expert in my own life experience. Over the past twenty years I have sought guidance from a myriad of healers and alternative therapists and practitioners in hopes of unlocking the secret to true health and happiness. I studied holistic nutrition at the Institute for Integrative Nutrition in New York in order to better understand what healthy eating truly means. I have studied psychology, spirituality, quantum physics, energy medicine, ancient wisdom, and various forms of healing. And while I am a firm believer that diet and lifestyle are essential factors in staying healthy, I've also come to realize that our minds, and the thoughts and beliefs we hold, have a direct and powerful effect on our biology.

I'm convinced we have more power to heal than we've been led to believe. But you don't have to take my word for it—I've gone out on the road and interviewed leading scientists, doctors, and teachers in the fields of mind/ body medicine, such as Deepak Chopra, Bruce Lipton, Marianne Williamson, Michael B. Beckwith, Kelly Turner, and more.

Heal not only taps into these brilliant minds, but it also dives into incredible real-life healing journeys of people I've met along the way. Through these survivors' inspiring and emotional stories, we'll delve deeply into what worked, what didn't, and why. I feel strongly that learning about others' success stories bolsters and strengthens our belief in our own possibilities. Healing can be extremely complex and deeply personal, and it can happen for a variety of reasons. It can even happen spontaneously.

The intention of this book is to flip on the switch of awareness, illuminating what's really at the root of the chronic illness epidemic and what is truly possible when it comes to healing. The latest science reveals that we are not always victims of unchangeable genes, nor should we buy into a scary prognosis. The fact is we have more control over our health and life than we have been taught to believe. This book will empower you with a new understanding of the miraculous human body and the extraordinary healing potential within us all.

Let's begin.

What Is Health?

Natural forces within us are the true healers of disease.

—Hippocrates

Too many of us feel powerless when it comes to our health. We have been taught by modern society that we are victims of our genes, at the mercy of a random (or predestined) fate, and the only ones who can save us are doctors in white coats, with their stethoscopes, scalpels, and prescription pads of miracles. But are pills and surgeries really the best solutions to treat the increasing prevalence of chronic illness and disease?

With almost half of the United States suffering from a chronic illness,[1] the answer is proving to be more multi-faceted than simply prescribing a pill or scheduling surgery. A chronic condition is defined as one that is persistent, recurring, or otherwise long-lasting in its effects—a disease that comes with time. The term *chronic* is often applied when the course of the disease lasts for more than three months and can be distinguished from a condition that is termed acute (sudden in onset and typically more severe). It is important to distinguish between an acute illness and a chronic illness, because as you will discover in this book, one of the main issues with our declining health and failing healthcare system is that we are applying an acute medical model to chronic illnesses, and we are falling short of getting to the root causes and achieving lasting healing.

Science and technology have advanced more rapidly over the past century than ever before, yet we are sicker and more depressed than ever. Cancer, a chronic illness, has become far too prevalent and is just as terrifying a diagnosis as it was forty years ago. Anxiety and depression seem as common as a cold, and autoimmune diseases are spreading like a heat rash in the summer.

What is going on? Has our world become so toxic that illness is inevitable? While the chemicals in processed food and our household products can certainly contribute to disease, *Heal* is not another book about diet, nutrition, and green living. *This is a book about how deeply connected our minds are to our biology, and the tremendous effect our thoughts, beliefs, and emotions have on our physical health.*

"Do the best you can until you know better.
Then when you know better, you do better."

—Maya Angelou

The Impact of Stress

What is health? Among its definitions for *health*, the *Merriam-Webster Collegiate Dictionary* lists:

> The condition of being sound in body, mind, or spirit, *especially*: freedom from physical disease or pain; a condition in which someone or something is thriving or doing well: well-being.

If health is freedom from physical "dis-ease," then we might say that health is actually a state of *ease*. We might also assume that thriving, or good health, should be our natural state, just as we see flowers blooming and thriving in the wild without having to "do" anything. It follows, then, that when we get sick, we should ask ourselves what might be knocking us out of balance or out of our natural state of thriving? According to experts, the biggest culprit is stress.

The Scary Truth about Stress

I've been in practice for thirty-five years now, and I've seen a lot of patients. I've seen a lot of crazy things, and I'm more firmly convinced every week that goes by that the ultimate cause of disease is stress.

—**Dr. Jeffrey Thompson**

Ninety percent of what takes people to the doctor is stress-related illness—but they leave with antidepressants; they leave with every kind of medication.

—**Joan Borysenko, PhD**

We have three basic stresses. We have physical stress, like accidents, injuries, falls, or traumas. We have chemical stress, like bacteria, viruses, hormones in foods, heavy metals, hangovers, and blood sugar levels. And then we have emotional stress, like family tragedies, loss, job, or finances. All of those things knock our brain and body out of balance.

—**Dr. Joe Dispenza**

In this age of information we are constantly inundated with bad news, under tremendous pressure to "keep up with the Joneses," and experiencing a declining connection with the natural rhythms and cycles of the universe. All of these factors lead to enormous emotional stress. According to a 2016 article in *Time* magazine, the post-9/11 generation has been "raised in an era of economic and national insecurity. They've never known a time when terrorism and school shootings weren't the norm. They grew up watching their parents weather a severe recession, and, perhaps most important, they hit puberty at a time when technology and social media were transforming society."[2]

Incidents of depression and anxiety in teenagers are skyrocketing because of the heartbreaking pressures of social media and an ever-increasing competitive culture to achieve. Social, political, and environmental causes are likely implicated in an increase in the number of teens each year who have had a depressive episode—up 37 percent between 2005 and 2014.[3] High school students today have more anxiety symptoms and are twice as likely to see a mental health professional as teens in the 1980s.[4] This is great for drug companies that produce antidepressants and ADHD medication. Not so great for the developing minds and bodies of our children.

Along with the rise of emotional stressors, we are experiencing a parallel rise of chemical stressors in modern society. Because of the bulk and convenience trends in the food industry,

- we are seeing more cheap chemical substitutes and preservatives in our food;
- we are eating out-of-season, nonlocal food that is often picked in another country and flash-ripened with gas after two weeks in transit to its destination;
- we are consuming genetically modified produce and animal products from animals being fed unnatural diets, hormones, and antibiotics, which can have a detrimental effect on whoever consumes them.

According to the Center for Food Safety, "It has been estimated that upwards of 75 percent of processed foods on supermarket shelves—from soda to soup, crackers to condiments—contain genetically engineered ingredients."[5] These food-like substances and chemical stressors amount to a detrimental burden on our bodies. Our digestive systems get confused and sick, and our immune systems can't keep up with their detox, repair, and regenerate functions. Also, in addition to our foods, harmful chemicals in many cleaning and beauty products are disrupting our hormones and adding to the tremendous toxic burden on our bodies. As we move further away from natural ingredients and real food, we move further away from our natural state of health.

As our immune systems become taxed and overwhelmed by the modern onslaught of emotional and chemical stresses, we become more susceptible to bacteria, viruses, and other pathogens in our environments. It has become clear that our conveniently plastic-wrapped modern lifestyle is a double-edged sword. So how can we take the best of what science and technology has to offer, yet protect ourselves from the negative side effects of some advancements? The answer is found inside of us.

. . . .

How Modern Stress Manifests

When you perceive a threat . . . in the old days we referred to that as activating the adrenal system: fight or flight. If you're being chased by a saber-toothed tiger, how much energy do you want to make available to run away from that tiger? I hope you get the answer right! The answer is: I want 100 percent of the energy to run away from the tiger.

—Bruce Lipton, PhD

Centuries—thousands of years ago—fight or flight was appropriate because there was literally a life-threatening situation with a wild animal. But now it's your spouse or your boss or rent that's due in a week, and yet the system reacts in the same way, as though it's a life-threatening situation. So you're still releasing cortisol, adrenaline, and noradrenaline into the system.

—**Peter Crone**

If you're running a fight-or-flight response all the time, by definition, you are mobilizing resources from your gut, from your elimination system, from your immune system, from your higher brain centers, and putting that energy into your muscles to fight for your life. That means your memory is not all that good, your concentration is down, you can't digest your food properly, you can't eliminate toxins properly, and your immune system is compromised, chronically, all the time.

—**Dr. Jeffrey Thompson**

• •

The body's stress response is designed for a sprint—fight or flight to save your life—but these days we are all running a chronic stress marathon. If we don't allow ourselves the opportunity to fall back into a state of rest and repair, we put our health at risk. Finding ways to manage daily stress, whether it's exercise, meditation, a walk outside, or simply powering down from technology, will help you feel calm and centered and let your body recharge, repair, and return to a state of ease.

Are you running a daily stress marathon? Do you give yourself time to rest and repair?

What are two daily practices you can commit to in order to manage your stress?

As a child I remember being so fascinated by the body's ability to heal. When I scraped my knee, my mom would clean the cut, shower it with kisses, and then leave it to heal all by itself. It seemed so magical at the time that in a matter of days my knee would be as good as new, with little or no evidence that a scrape ever existed. We've lost sight of the body's incredible, innate ability to heal because we have been conditioned by society to believe that we need a doctor to save us or give us an external remedy to restore health.

Every television show or movie I can remember watching in my childhood involved a man in a white coat coming to the house with a little black bag full of lifesaving remedies when someone was ill. Nowadays, shows tend to focus on lifesaving drama in the emergency room. All of these images have taught us that when we are sick or injured we need something or someone outside of ourselves in order to heal. Doctors possess the ability to set a broken bone, but it is the natural intelligence built into the DNA of every cell that actually regenerates and heals the bone. A loving mother or father may disinfect a scrape, but it is the natural intelligence and function of the immune system that rebuilds, regenerates, and ultimately heals the tissue.

But does this same healing power apply to more complex chronic conditions such as cancer, autoimmune illness, and mental health issues such as depression or Alzheimer's? This very question is a big part of what motivated me to embark on this healing exploration and seek answers from experts. How deep does our innate healing power really go?

. . . .

Our Natural Intelligence

You have an egg and a sperm, and they come together. Then these cells start emerging. They start dividing and collaborating and become brains, bones, eyeballs, fingers, toes, hearts, and livers. There is a natural intelligence that leads those cells from an embryo to a baby. There's a natural intelligence that leads an acorn into an oak tree. There's a natural intelligence that keeps the planets revolving around the sun. That same natural intelligence continues to work in your body. Right at this moment your lungs are breathing and your heart is beating.

—**Marianne Williamson**

The intelligence that's giving us life, that's keeping our heart beating and digesting our food and runs through the autonomic nervous system—it's the greatest healer in the world. All we have to do is get out of the way.

—**Dr. Joe Dispenza**

. . . .

As modern society advances, we are moving further and further away from nature and the natural rhythm, function, and order of things. We need to find the right balance of incorporating ancient wisdom and natural medicine, while utilizing the best and least harmful technological advancements science has to offer. Nature, with its immensely complex beauty, unfolds perfectly until something artificial or man-made gets in the way. Nature keeps itself in balance, self-regulates, regenerates, and self-cleans. The human body is the same. Our bodies are designed to self-regulate and heal. Technology (electrical and chemical) and fearful consciousness (inadequacy, greed, and the illusion of separation) are what's getting in the way. It is time to merge new science with ancient wisdom and reestablish the harmony and balance that is so evident in nature.

> "Man's chief delusion is his conviction
> that there are *causes other than his own
> state of consciousness.*"
> **—Neville Goddard**

· ·

You Are the Architect of Your Own Healing

The best science of our time is now showing that every organ in the human body has the ability to heal itself, given the right environment. Even the organs we were told could not, like spinal cord tissue, brain tissue, heart tissue, pancreatic tissue, and prostate tissue. All of these organs are actually designed to repair and heal themselves under the right conditions, given the right environment. What are those conditions? That's the question. Some of them are environmental, things like water, air, and the quality of our food. Some of them may be chemical, like the supplements that we take and some of the herbal products our ancestors understood and used with great success in healing their bodies before modern medicine ever came along. And I think those are interesting, but what really fascinates me is the inner environment. This is the environment that the Buddha talked to us about so eloquently when he said that every man and woman is the architect of their own healing and their own destiny.

—**Gregg Braden**

· ·

The mind-body connection is the "inner environment" that Gregg Braden speaks of—perhaps one of the most important factors in the health of our bodies. Our outer environment and the lifestyle choices we make—the food we eat, the water we drink, and the air we breathe—all play an important role in our overall health. But when it comes to healing, perhaps the most important factors are the thoughts in our minds and the emotions in our hearts.

"Your body is simply a living expression of your point of view of the world."

—**Carl Frederick**

Modern medicine has barely begun to incorporate the new science that proves the mind's effect on the body. In this book we will discover how our thoughts, beliefs, and emotions affect our health, perhaps to an even greater degree than diet and exercise, or even a prescription. We will learn that the body really *is* designed to heal itself and how to activate the powerful healing mechanism within. We will take our health back into our own hands.

Conventional medicine has its place, and I'm grateful to live in an age when we know so much about the physical human body. But until we've uncovered the truth about how the mind-body connection really works, we remain power-less victims in a scary world. The mind and body are deeply connected, and *all* of us are deeply connected to the world around us. So much more is possible when it comes to heal-ing our bodies than we are being led to believe, and we can reveal these truths to make empowered choices and live life to the fullest every day.

Our bodies are not only designed to heal, we are meant to thrive and, as you will discover, the answers are within you.

"There are only two days in the year that nothing can be done. One is called yesterday and the other is called tomorrow. Today is the right day to love, believe, do, and mostly live."

—His Holiness the Dalai Lama

Chapter 1 Takeaways

- It's time to address the prevalence of chronic disease and make changes that support our natural state of health and ease.
- Ninety percent of what brings people to the doctor is stress-related illness.
- There are three basic types of stress: physical, chemical, and emotional—all of which can knock our bodies out of balance.
- Our bodies possess a natural intelligence that keeps us alive, self-regulating and regenerating without us even thinking about it.
- Our thoughts, beliefs, and emotions have an extremely powerful effect on our physical health.
- We need to take charge of our health, seek out ways to tap into our mind-body connection, and activate the powerful healer within us all.

Your Body Is Not a Machine

If you want to find the secrets of the universe,
think in terms of energy, frequency, and vibration.
—**Nikola Tesla**

The quality of healthcare, especially in the United States, is rapidly declining. Costs are going up, and overall wellness is going down. According to the National Health Council: "Chronic diseases affect approximately 133 million Americans, representing more than 40 percent of the total population of this country. By 2020, that number is projected to grow to an estimated 157 million, with 81 million having multiple conditions."[6] The Centers for Disease Control and Prevention estimate that chronic illness is the leading driver of the nation's $3.3 trillion in annual healthcare costs.[7]

Quite frankly, our modern medical model is failing us. But new sciences such as quantum physics and epigenetics have begun to prove that our bodies are more connected with our minds and emotions than conventional medicine has ever accounted for. What was once considered woo-woo is now being supported by these sciences. Healing modalities like acupuncture, sound healing, energy healing, and the use of herbs and food as medicine are still labeled as alternative, when in fact they have been in use and proven effective by our ancestors and their ancient traditions for thousands of years.

I spoke with Gregg Braden, one of the world's most spiritually influential people and a Templeton Prize nominee, about why our medical system is failing us. He said: "We say that science began about three hundred years ago when Isaac Newton formalized the laws of physics. These laws tell us that the origin of human life is random, that we are separate from our bodies, and essentially powerless when it comes to healing our bodies. They also tell us that we are separate from the world beyond our bodies. Not only do we have very little influence over what happens within, but we have no influence over what happens in the world beyond our bodies."

In 1859, Charles Darwin published *On the Origin of Species*, considered the foundation of evolutionary biology. Darwin claimed that nature is based upon a model of competition and conflict—natural selection. Greg had this to say: "Darwin's ideas of separation and competition are so deeply ingrained into our lives and our world today that we almost take them for granted." Gregg continued, "Darwin had no way of knowing in his time what we know today. He couldn't have known about cells and neurites and DNA that we only have discovered recently. We also now know that a field exists that connects all things. It's causing problems in the scientific community because the mathematics are based upon the absence of this field."

How has this negatively impacted modern medicine?

. . . .

Science Is Changing, and We Need to Catch Up

We are now about three centuries into a mind-set in medicine that was predicated on the work of Descartes, Newton, and Darwin even. This idea that our symptoms are meaningless, that our body is a machine full of organs with buttons and levers that need adjusting and that you're really not here for any purposeful existence, you're here to live and survive until you die.

—Kelly Brogan, MD

Medicine being derived from Newtonian physics looks at the body as a physical device, and if there's anything wrong with it, it is a consequence of a problem in the mechanics of a physical machine. I say this is really cool until 1925. In 1925, a new physics came along: quantum physics. What's the relevance of quantum physics? Well, it said that invisible energy that was out there, that we did not even talk about in medicine because we are just a physical body, it turns out that our perception of what is physical is an illusion. There's nothing physical at all, it's all energy.

A long, long time ago, the word *spirit* was what: invisible moving forces that influence the physical realm. Quantum physics is taking us back to a time that said the invisible forces that we have been discounting in medicine turn out to be the primary forces that control everything. And I say, "Well, what do they include?" Mind and consciousness. **And this is why if you want to come back to the supreme power over our biology, it's thought. That invisible energy from our mind that not only shapes our body but shapes our relationship to the world in which we live.**

—Bruce Lipton, PhD

The best science of the late twentieth and early twenty-first centuries has overturned three hundred years of scientific thinking with new discoveries that are peer-reviewed in the scientific literature. Science is now telling us that the fundamental rule of nature is actually based upon cooperation and not the competition and the conflict that Darwin proposed one hundred fifty years ago. Biologists call it mutual aid. The best science of our day is also telling us that we are deeply connected to our bodies, and that our thoughts, feelings, emotions, and beliefs that originate both in the brain and in the heart trigger the chemistry that can actually reverse disease, heal our bodies, and trigger longevity in ways that have not commonly been accepted in the West. Modern medicine is based upon the old ideas of separation, competition, and conflict on a biological level, on a cellular level, in our bodies.

—Gregg Braden

If you look inside any part of your body with a microscope, you look inside your hand, you find cells. You look inside the cells, you get your DNA in the center of the cell. You look inside the DNA, you find atoms. You look inside the atoms, there's nothing there. Well, there are protons, neutrons, and electrons. But what's amazing is that inside an atom, there's 99.9999999999999 percent empty space. If a proton was the size of an apple, the closest electron would be the size of a grain of salt and it'd be approximately two kilometers away. Now, that's how much space you would get; simple pi r squared [πr^2]. The particles themselves, they actually emerge essentially out of what's called the quantum field and ultimately, you can think of particles as just waves of energy. They are just literally vibrations of energy, and I think it shifts your mind from thinking that something is seemingly solid and permanent to perhaps something can change and something can be healed.

—**David R. Hamilton, PhD**

. . . .

With new discoveries in science, such as quantum physics and epigenetics, it is imperative that we adapt the way we look at our own biology. In the study of quantum physics, science is now proving that we are connected through a field, and all matter is actually made up of vibrating waves of energy that can shift through the influence of thought and intention. New findings in epigenetics are demonstrating that we are not simply victims of our genes, but that our genes are just a blueprint, and we can activate or deactivate them based on our thoughts, emotions, and lifestyle choices. Our current conventional medical model is not yet taking into account that these new sciences are demonstrating how everything is energy, how everything in our bodies and outside our bodies is connected, and how our thoughts, beliefs, emotions, and lifestyle choices influence our biology.

Holistic Medicine

When we discuss conventional medicine versus holistic medicine, it's important to understand what *holistic* really means, because there continues to be a stigma attached to that label. Many people believe holistic medicine is not based on science and proper research. The term *holistic* simply means that we are looking to treat and heal the complete system rather than the individual parts. Holistic medicine accounts for both the mind and the entire body, as opposed to specialized or compartmentalized medicine, which may treat just one organ system or part without taking into account the *whole* organism.

As a philosophy, holistic is also characterized as a sum of its parts, interconnected and explained only by the entire system. Holistic medicine, therefore, considers a person's mental, emotional, and social factors, not just their physical symptoms. This is why so many people find holistic medicine both effective and compassionate, because they often feel less like a patient and more like a human being. Now that experts agree that our bodies and minds are intricately connected, and that we are deeply connected to each other and our environment, it makes logical sense that holistic medicine is a more effective way to approach our best health.

· ·

Why Conventional Medicine Isn't Always Effective

We are in an awkward transition now because we're bumping up against the limitations of a model of medicine that may have served us for a window of time. The types of illnesses that patients are presenting with today are complex, and they cannot be addressed in a twenty-minute appointment with a family practice doctor who doesn't have the training or wherewithal to dive deep into the interconnectedness between multiple different systems that we were always taught are discrete and separate.

—Kelly Brogan, MD

We have a sick care system where doctors and insurance companies are basically treating symptoms but aren't really getting to root causes, and in many cases aren't dealing with the whole person. They're dealing with the symptom by giving a drug, which then has a

side effect, and so it keeps on spinning—more toxicity, more disease, and more ill health.

—**Dr. Michael B. Beckwith**

You've got to get to the root cause of your disease
if you're going to find freedom. People are looking
to solutions without looking at, "Why do I have the
problem in the first place?"

—**Peter Crone**

Conventional medicine is tied up in an old belief system and locked in to the cause of illness being tied
into our genetics and our biochemistry, and therefore the pharmaceutical industry is the great savior.
Why? Because it'll make the chemistry that should
bring us back to health again. Well, it turns out that's
totally false. There are so few diseases that are actually organic. In fact, 100 percent of type 2 diabetes has
nothing to do with genetics and everything to do with
lifestyle. Ninety percent or more of cardiovascular
disease has nothing organically wrong with the individual; it's just a consequence of dealing with stress.

—**Bruce Lipton, PhD**

Almost anyone can reverse type 2 diabetes with lifestyle changes in a month's time, and it will simply go

away. Get rid of the carbs and start to exercise. Get rid of the junk food. Eat whole foods with low carbs, and your whole insulin sensitivity is going to reset itself. This is what we can do for ourselves. **That's why chronic illnesses are really opportunities for lifestyle change and change of mind.**

—Joan Borysenko, PhD

. . . .

Your Body as Communicator

We aren't only a community of human cells. We are actually a superorganism made up of trillions of human cells *and* microbes. Microbes are microorganisms like bacteria that actually play an essential role in all of our bodily functions and make up what is called our microbiome.

Bruce Lipton explained what the microbiome is and how it works: "Today we find that there are as many microbes, bacteria, parasites in our body as human cells. Are they invaders? The answer is *no*. We cannot live without them. If you remove the bacteria, called the microbiome, which is the community of bacteria that live within us, you will die. The bacteria are not an adjunct to our life; they're required for a life. The microbiome, the bacteria in your body, is required for your digestion and running your entire system.

There's a feedback between the bacteria and genes of your own body. They're in community."

Not only do we have communication between the microbiome and our human cells, but we also have communication between our cells and the environment, or the world around us. Have you ever gotten chills and the hair on your arms stands on end? This can happen when adrenaline is released in the body as a result of feeling threatened or cold. It can also indicate a reaction to coherent or incoherent frequencies, or what are commonly referred to as good or bad vibes in your environment. All of these electrical and chemical feedback systems are in place for our survival.

Another one of these brilliant feedback mechanisms is the symptom. Symptoms are evidence of an imbalance going on beneath the surface. They are a conversation our body is trying to have with us, or a warning bell to alert us that something is off that needs our attention. One of the problems with Western medicine is that our first action is usually to get rid of or suppress the symptoms with medication, in order to give the patient some immediate relief.

"Symptoms are like a smoke alarm going off to get my attention. When a smoke alarm goes off and starts to try to get my attention, the final approach of a treatment should not be to silence the smoke alarm, but to put out the fire that caused the smoke."

—Dr. Jeffrey Thompson

The modern medical model is based on specialization. One can be a specialist in dermatology, neurology, anesthesiology, surgery, pediatrics, pathology, stem cell biology, and so on. The problem with educating our doctors in a specialized manner is that they look at symptoms from the perspective and language of their specialty, often without respect for the fact that every cell, organ, and system in the human body is part of an intricate community designed to work together in order to adapt, self-regulate, and heal. When you treat only one specific area of the body, that drug, surgical intervention, or other conventional treatment will throw off the function and communication of the entire system.

. . . .

Is Modern Medicine Still Useful?

Does this mean medicine's all negative? Absolutely not. Medicine does miracles with trauma. If I physically hurt myself—I get in a car accident and my guts are hanging out—don't send me to a chiropractor. And I don't need a massage therapist, and homeopathy is really not going to help. I want a surgeon.

—**Bruce Lipton, PhD**

Medicine is useful. Pharmaceutical medicine, therapeutic interventions, surgery, etc., are useful, I would say, in acute illnesses. Otherwise, if you have a chronic illness, doesn't matter what it is—cancer, heart disease, autoimmune illnesses—use a holistic approach, which means everything from mind, body, emotions, energy healing, even distant healing— anything that influences your experiences of mind, body, emotions.

—**Deepak Chopra, MD**

Less than 5 percent of the people on the planet are born with [fully penetrant] genetic conditions. The other 95 percent, their diseases are created from lifestyle and behaviors and choices. So the medical model works really great for acute conditions—like if you break your arm or you have appendicitis, it's a good idea to seek emergency medical care. But when it comes to chronic conditions that require a lifestyle change, a lot of times it's not enough just to take a chemical.

—**Dr. Joe Dispenza**

What we have done is take emergency management and applied it to chronic care, and this is why half of Americans are taking as many as five prescriptions and still feeling unwell. The analogy we use in functional medicine is that if you have a piece of glass stuck in your foot, you can put a Band-Aid over it, sure. You can take a Tylenol for it, but it certainly makes a lot more sense to just figure out how to take it out, right?

—**Kelly Brogan, MD**

. . . .

A fully penetrant genetic condition means that if you have a certain gene or genetic mutation, the disease or condition will be expressed 100 percent of the time, regardless of lifestyle choices. Drs. Chopra, Dispenza, and Lipton all agree that fully penetrant conditions make up approximately 5 percent of the world's population, which means that 95 percent of us have the power to impact our own health through our lifestyle choices. If you are dealing with a genetic disorder, it is a good idea to ask your doctor about the penetrance of your condition. If it is not fully penetrant, you have some influence and control over the expression of the disease. Once we believe that our diet, thoughts, emotions, stress levels, sleep quality, and so forth all play a role in our well-being and physical health, we can seek out doctors and practitioners who will take these factors into account and treat us as whole people. Naturopathic medicine, lifestyle medicine, integrative medicine, and functional medicine are examples of fields that look at—and treat—the patient as a whole person. Again, conventional treatments and pharmaceutical medicine aren't all negative. Sometimes we must weigh the consequences and elect to do a life-saving procedure or treatment at the expense of the optimal function of the entire system, in order to simply survive. We are extremely fortunate to live in an age where we have access to incredible lifesaving technology. But those modalities should mostly be used in acute, emergency situations. Chronic illness requires a look into the mental, emotional, spiritual, and physical aspects of our lives.

Is your doctor treating you as a whole person? If you are seeing specialists, do they take into account how their specific area of expertise is connected to and interacts with all the other systems of the body? Are they taking into account things like diet, stress, and emotional state?

The Energy of Water

A Japanese scientist named Dr. Masaru Emoto did some fascinating research with water and frequency in the 1990s. In 2008, Dr. Emoto published his findings in the *Journal of Scientific Exploration*, a peer-reviewed scientific journal of the Society for Scientific Exploration. Dr. Emoto took bottles of water and placed intentions into the water by physically labeling the bottles with different words. For example, he labeled one bottle of water "hate" and labeled another bottle of water "love." Upon freezing samples of the water from each of the bottles, Dr. Emoto discovered that the frozen love water formed as beautiful, perfectly symmetrical crystals. The crystals of the hate water were disjointed and abnormal looking. You can see images of these experiments in Dr. Emoto's book, *The Hidden Messages in Water*, or view them online at www.masaru-emoto.net.

Masaru also demonstrated that water exposed to the words "thank you" formed beautiful symmetrical crystals, no matter what the language, while water exposed to "you fool" and other degrading words resulted in disjointed, broken crystals. "The entire universe is in a state of vibration, and each thing generates its own frequency, which is unique," Emoto explains.[8] "Water—so sensitive to the unique frequencies being emitted by the world—essentially and efficiently mirrors the outside world."[9]

The reason I think this is incredibly significant is that our bodies are made up of 70 percent water. Dr. Emoto's work shows us that the energy and intention of our environment directly affects the health and function of our bodies. Energy and thoughts have the ability to change the frequency of our blood, our cells, and our tissues. This is why I believe negative self-talk stemming from disempowering beliefs like "I am not enough" can affect our physical health. So many of us beat ourselves up and call ourselves degrading words when we aren't the perfect weight, or we make a mistake, or we are betrayed in a relationship. Can you imagine the effect our negative thoughts and self-talk have on our cells, based on Emoto's research? It further implies that the frequencies of love and gratitude are healing and aligned with nature, while negative frequencies like hate or fear can have a damaging or dis-ease effect.

While his experiments may be controversial, Dr. Emoto's findings confirm for me that thoughts and intentions really do affect body matter.

"Water is the mirror that has the ability to show us what we cannot see. It is the blueprint for our reality, which can change with a single, positive thought."

—**Dr. Masaru Emoto**

Radical Remission

Radical (or spontaneous) remission is when a person heals from cancer against all odds, or when it is statistically unexpected. Kelly Turner, PhD, a Harvard-educated cancer researcher, has studied radical remissions for more than ten years. It began with a trip around the world to interview radical remission survivors from all different countries, and the fascinating healers who helped them achieve that remission. Since then, she's analyzed over 1,500 of these cases and conducted more than 250 in-depth interviews with radical remission survivors from all walks of life, every race, every religion, every age, and most important, every cancer type. She wrote about her discoveries in her groundbreaking book, *Radical Remission*.

"Radical remissions have been verified and reported for every single cancer type," Kelly told me. "It's tremendously hopeful to know that—even people with pancreatic cancer, stage IV lung cancer, or even a brain tumor that's considered inoperable—there are examples of people out there who have healed from it. Does that mean that we're all going to heal tomorrow? No. But it means they deserve to be studied, and there's something incredible there for us to learn."

"In all, " Kelly said, "I've discovered over seventy-five different things that people have done to try to get well. But not everybody uses all seventy-five of these healing factors. However, when I looked closer at the data, they were all using the same nine factors. They came up with [these factors]; I just listened. Of the nine factors that radical remission survivors are using, only two of them are physical. The rest are mental, emotional, and spiritual. And that hit me like a ton of bricks. So, there really is a way to activate the immune system with your mental, emotional work. And, of course, there is plenty of science behind that."

The Nine Key Factors to Radical Remission

1. Radically changing your diet
2. Taking control of your health
3. Following your intuition
4. Using herbs and supplements
5. Releasing suppressed emotions
6. Increasing positive emotions
7. Embracing social support
8. Deepening your spiritual connection
9. Having strong reasons for living

I believe that while Kelly Turner's research applies only to cancer, these nine essential factors can apply to healing all types of chronic conditions. I also find it so compelling that out of the nine key factors, only two of them are physical. This exemplifies for me that if we want to heal or achieve optimal health, only about 20 percent of the equation is physical, while perhaps the most important parts of the formula are the mental, emotional, and spiritual work. Kelly's research is just more confirmation for me why a holistic approach to healing is the most effective path when it comes to chronic illness. One remarkable example of radical remission that demonstrates how powerful the mental, emotional, and spiritual aspects are when it comes to healing is Anita Moorjani's story. She is living proof that no matter how far gone the body seems, it is possible for tissues to regenerate, function to restore, and the body to heal.

Anita Moorjani's Story

February 2, 2006, should have been the last day of Anita Moorjani's life. Four years prior, with just a lump on her neck, she had been diagnosed with lymphoma. Now, she had tumors, some of them the size of lemons, from the base of her skull, all around her neck, under her arms, in her chest, and all the way down to her abdomen. She was so weak that her organs were shutting down one by one and she went into a coma. The doctors told her family that these were her final hours.

Anita recounted to me that while she was in the coma she went into another realm where she became aware of her deceased father:

When I was growing up, my father and I had a very turbulent relationship. As a teenager and a young woman my parents wanted to gear me up for an arranged marriage, which is very normal in my Hindu culture. But because I grew up in a Hong

Kong school that taught British values, I didn't want to have an arranged marriage, so I rebelled against their wishes. I was always left with this feeling that I had let my father down and that I had never been the kind of daughter he wanted me to be. Now here I was, with him in the other realm, and all I felt from him and for him was pure, unconditional love. There was no judgment from him at all for anything that I had done. In that moment I reached a state of complete and total clarity, and in that state of clarity I understood why I had the cancer. I understood how it was that every decision and every choice I had made in my life up to that point was made from fear.

Now that Anita knew this truth, she realized that if she chose to go back to her body, it would heal. But even still, she didn't want to go back to her body. The immense love she felt in this other realm, and the connection she was having with her father, felt too good. But her father told her she must go back and fulfill her purpose, and it was in those moments that she felt herself coming out of the coma. It is important to note that while she was in the coma, Anita was aware of things she couldn't possibly have perceived in her state. When she woke up from the coma, she recalled the doctor's name who attended to her in the coma, whom she hadn't met before, and she described in detail what the nurses had done to her while she lay there unconscious. She also recounted a conversation her husband and her doctor had about forty feet down the hall, well out of earshot.

After about a week out of the coma, the doctors could actually see that Anita's tumors were dissolving faster than they'd ever seen tumors dissolve before. At the end of five weeks, Anita was physically stronger and they could find no trace of cancer in her body, so they let her go home and live her life—cancer-free. Anita has all of the medical records proving what happened to her physically.

During Anita's near-death experience, she made a dramatic shift in the way she looked at life. She went from viewing life through a lens of fear—fear of judgment, fear of what other people think, fear of failure, and so on—to shifting her perception to one of love. Her body responded to her change in consciousness and it healed. Remarkable! It is important to note that Anita had done chemotherapy and sought out other Western interventions earlier on her journey; however by the time she went into a coma and had the near-death experience she was in such a bad state that her doctors were preparing her family to say their good-byes. The only thing that changed between that state and a healed one was her perception of life. But is Anita's case a random miracle or can we study what happened to her, so that more of us can achieve this incredible transformation?

Chapter 2 Takeaways

- Science is evolving, and we must adapt our thinking beyond the idea that the body is simply a physical device.
- Holistic medicine considers a person's mental, emotional, and lifestyle factors, not just their physical symptoms. Now that the experts agree that our bodies and minds are intricately connected, and that we are deeply connected to each other and our environment, it makes logical sense that a holistic approach is vitally important to our health and well-being.
- The body is brilliantly made up of a community of human cells and a larger microbiome that are constantly interacting to adapt, self-regulate, and heal.
- Conventional, specialized treatment of symptoms can throw off the function and communication of the entire system.
- Radical remissions have been seen in people all over the world, with every type of cancer.
- There are nine key factors all survivors have used to heal themselves, and only two of them are physical. The rest are mental, emotional, and spiritual.

The Power of Your Subconscious Mind

The mind is everything. What you think you become.

—widely attributed to Buddha

Anita Moorjani changed nothing but her perception of life, and her body responded and healed. She achieved a feat that her doctors and loved ones believed was impossible based on the advanced deterioration of her physical body. How we interpret the world is based on our beliefs about life, and it is often said that there are two types of people. Some wear the metaphorical "rose-colored glasses" and have a positive outlook on life. Some are pessimists and look at life through a darker, more cynical lens. The color of our perception is determined by our core belief systems, most of which we establish in early childhood.

. . . .

When Our Beliefs Begin

When we look at the world, we're actually operating through the subconscious mind. The programs in your subconscious mind primarily came from downloading other people's behaviors—your mother, your father, your siblings, and your community—in the first seven years of life. Most of the programs, 70 percent or so, are negative, disempowering, and self-sabotaging.

—**Bruce Lipton, PhD**

We were essentially an open sponge to the world, absorbing the patterns from all of those people that we were exposed to and surrounded with at a young age. So, if we had caregivers who were really conscious and learned to manage their emotions and heal their hurts in a healthy way, that's a really good thing. However, very few people I know were blessed enough to come from those families.

—**Gregg Braden**

Early conditioning influences everything from thought to emotions, perception to biology. If a child is receiving a lot of attention, affection, appreciation, acceptance, love, joy, then that will create biology that is self-regulating, homeostatic, and healthy. On the other hand, if the child is not given that acceptance, affection, or appreciation, that creates a feeling of separation and maybe fear. That ultimately will express itself as maybe anger, hostility, resentment, grievances, guilt, shame, or depression—and that creates separation. It's almost a cliché now; you have love on the one hand and fear on the other. Love is being connected to life, and fear is being disconnected. That fear is the base of all the other dysfunctional emotions I mentioned that create a disruption of homeostasis, of self-regulation, which then we say *dis-ease*, because it starts with discomfort but then becomes disease.

—**Deepak Chopra, MD**

Beliefs influence our perception. **We don't perceive truth; we perceive what we believe.** Now, certain beliefs can be really empowering, life affirming, and influence our greatest self. At the other end of the spectrum, there can be core, limiting beliefs, which ultimately are simply memories of a moment that haven't been fully formed because we're not able to process that moment. Let's say we're growing up in an environment where there's trauma in the household, alcoholism, or inflamed relationships. When we don't have tools to process our emotions in a given moment, we create a memory that's not fully formed. We don't integrate it, and it becomes a core, limiting belief. That core, limiting belief creates three things: one, a lens of perception; two, a filter for how we take in life; and three, a gravity or attractor field. We end up seeing ourselves and the world around us as if we're still four years old, in an environment of conflict, trauma, and drama. We filter and feel it every time colors, sounds, smells, tastes trigger our feelings. We then react as if that memory were going on for the first time. Furthermore, what we feel is what we attract.

So, you can attempt to outrun the subconscious mind, just like you attempt to outrun a shadow. You can't; you've got to turn around and face it. You've got to see the problem as the portal and recognize that these symptoms and stressors are meaningful and brilliantly intelligent in waking us up.

—**Dr. Darren Weissman**

. . . .

There are three important things to remember: first, most of our subconscious programming comes from other people (they aren't even our own beliefs!). Next, approximately 70 percent of our core belief systems happen to be negative and disempowering. Finally, when we don't have the tools to process emotions, our emotions get trapped in our subconscious mind and body as a memory that's not fully formed.

The term *subconscious* means to exist or operate in the mind beneath or beyond consciousness. In other words, we are often not even aware of the beliefs that are running our lives! Dr. Darren Weissman encourages us to see problems and circumstances in our lives as feedback or a portal to our subconscious mind. Our issues are meant to make us aware of our limiting and negative subconscious beliefs so that we can wake up and change the things that no longer serve us.

"When you change the way you look at things,
the things you look at change."

—Dr. Wayne Dyer

• •

The Early Evolution of Epigenetics

Back in 1968, I was learning how to clone stem cells, and at that time just a handful of people in the entire world even knew what a stem cell was, so I was in the right place at the right time to make some interesting discoveries. I put one stem cell in a culture by itself, and it divides every ten or twelve hours. At first, there's one, then two, four, eight, sixteen, thirty-two, doubling, until I eventually have fifty thousand genetically identical cells. But that's not the experiment, this is: I split the cells into three different petri dishes, and what I do is I change the chemical composition of the culture medium. Culture medium is the equivalent of blood. So, if I'm growing mouse cells, then what I do is look at mouse blood, see what it's made out of, and then try to make a synthetic version of that called culture medium. So I had genetically identical cells in three dishes, but each had slightly different environments because of the chemistry. In one dish the cells form muscle, in the second dish the cells form bone, and in the third dish the cells form fat cells. So, what controls the fate of the genetically identical cells? The environment was selecting the genetic activity of the cells.

The nature of biology is simple. Biological organisms adapt their biology to fit into an environment. Let's say I am looking at the activity of my liver cells in the body and I say, "Well, my liver cells should be adjusting 'to what's going on in the environment,'" and I say, "Well, how does the liver cell 'know what's going on in the environment?'" The answer is this: The liver cell is not touching the environment. It depends on the nervous system to send information about the environment inside the body, so the cells adjust their biology to match what's going on in the world. Well, we only have one problem with that. Consciousness is an interpretation. So, the mind reads the environment, makes an interpretation of the environment, and the brain translates that interpretation into the chemistry of the blood.

Therefore, my interpretation of life is what determines the chemical composition of my culture medium, my blood. That is what determines my genetics. As I change my thought, I change the chemistry. So, if I change my perception, my mind, change my belief about life, I change the signals that are going in and adjusting the function of the cell.

The point is very, very significant! I, by my ability to change my environment and by my ability to change my perception of the environment, have the ability to control my genetic activity. I'm not a victim of my heredity; I'm a master of my genetic activity.

—Bruce Lipton, PhD

• •

This book's message is about taking our health back into our own hands and realizing the incredible, innate ability our body has to heal. Dr. Lipton reminds us that consciousness is an interpretation, which is based on our beliefs about life that we adopted from our caregivers until seven years old.

As we saw in Anita's case, her core beliefs were based in fear, which theoretically led to stress, turmoil, and eventually disease. As soon as she experienced the clarity and the unconditional love from and for her father during her near-death experience, her core beliefs shifted to being based in love and her body naturally went back into a state of ease and health. Our perception of life, based on our beliefs, determines how we see the world—either through a rose-colored, empowered lens or a darker, negative lens. This lens or filter is what ultimately determines our level of emotional stress. And remember what almost all the experts stated in chapter 1: stress—whether chemical, emotional, or physical—is at the root of almost all dis-ease.

. . . .

The Power of Belief

People who have the same DNA, who have the same susceptibility to illness, one can become ill and the other can stay well. One can heal and the other can't. All because they optimize the environmental factors that control gene activity, and that is what the field of epigenetics is all about.

—Joan Borysenko, PhD

Stress that most people have psychologically is fictitious. It's made up about a potentially worst-case scenario and future event that hasn't happened yet. Stress like that is occurring when we're resisting life. There's something in life that we say we don't want or it should be different or they shouldn't do that, and we're creating our own stress. We're not in harmony with life and not accepting life. That's what will create a lack of ease, which is why I love the word *dis-ease*. So the lack of ease is the precursor to disease, which then obviously gets manifested in our physiology.

My specialty is working with the mind and helping people see where they're stuck within beliefs of inadequacy. That, for me, is usually a precursor to their suffering. Suffering then stimulates the chemical shit storm that goes on in their body that then degenerates their tissues, etc. Until you shift your mind-set and belief about life, until you find true inner peace, then you can bombard any kind of disorder that you have, and chances are you may get rid of it for a sort of transitory period, but it's most likely going to come back.

—Peter Crone

The power of belief is almost everything. What you are believing and thinking at this moment is telling your immune system to either stop and not work because you have to run from a stressor, or it is saying, "Everything's cool, why don't we relax, and if there's anything that needs to be cleaned up, let's clean up." That's it. You're either in fight-or-flight [mode] or you're in rest-and-repair [mode], and it's your beliefs that toggle that switch.

—Kelly Turner, PhD

* * *

Is the lens through which you look at life positive and empowering or negative and disempowering? Do you feel like a helpless victim and that other people or outside circumstances are to blame for your problems? Or do you feel like you are a cocreator with life, and your thoughts, beliefs, and behaviors contribute to your experience? What are some subconscious beliefs that you hold that are coloring your lens? What are some of the beliefs that perhaps no longer serve you, and what are some new beliefs you would like to adopt?

"Although the world is full of suffering,
it is full also of the overcoming of it."

—Helen Keller

So how do we change our beliefs about life? How do we shift from fear to love? How do we learn how to process our emotions in a healthy way? Remember that about half of the people Kelly Turner studied (her research analyzed 1,500 cases of radical remission) were sent home to die because their conventional doctors could do nothing more to help them. These people healed by implementing variations of the nine key healing factors in chapter 2 (page 36). Many of these factors have to do with emotions, such as "*releasing suppressed emotions*" and "*increasing positive emotions.*"

Science is now proving that negative emotions such as rage, anger, hurt, fear, depression, and jealousy affect our biochemistry in a negative way. Positive emotions, on the other hand, cause our brains to release healing chemistry into our bodies, which boosts our immune systems. When we become aware of how our emotions affect our biology, we can start to implement practices or try different therapies that will help us to release suppressed emotions and increase positive emotions.

. . . .

The Impact of Emotions on Your Physiology

Before we get into too much talk about how you have to change your feelings and your thoughts, it's important to remember that this is rooted into the physical. So, your emotions and your spiritual connection are intimately tied to your physical body. We aren't just a physical body and then our brains are over here, thinking. They are together. They are one. If you make a change in one, there will be a change in the other, and we know that scientifically. When you're sent home on hospice, lying in bed and you can't go out and run half a mile, the one thing you can do is change your thoughts. And that's empowering.

—Kelly Turner, PhD

Every thought affects the body, as well as every other aspect of our lives because there is no separation between us. If I'm attacking you, I'm attacking myself. If I'm withholding compassion from you, I'm withholding compassion from myself, and that affects my body. You seek to forgive; you seek to have greater compassion as an act of self-interest. It's spiritual medicine. That's why the whole integrative approach to healing is the body, the mind, and the spirit. The mind literally affects the functioning of the immune system.

—**Marianne Williamson**

When we have an emotion within our heart, that emotion sends a signal to our brain. The quality of that signal determines what the brain does in response to the emotion. If you can imagine a signal from the heart to the brain that is a very smooth series of nice, even, coherent waves from the heart to the brain, the brain will match that smooth, even, organized chemistry and it will release chemistry that supports life in our bodies. This is where our immune systems become really strong and we have a super immune response. On the other hand, when we feel those moments of frustration, anger, hate, jealousy, rage, or fear, the signal looks different. It looks like a bad day on the stock market. It's a lot of very chaotic unorganized jagged waves going from the heart to the brain, and the brain receives those waves and says, "Oh, I need to match this chemistry." This is stress chemistry.

—**Gregg Braden**

When we're in a state of stress, our energy field goes into a state of resistance. That's why a polygraph works—we're able to read it. In that energy, our blood is affected and it doesn't flow as effectively. It heats up, cools down. When we're in stress, there's resistance, and it affects our pH. We become more acidic when we're in a state of stress. In a localized or systemic full-body acidity, inflammation occurs, which is just a reactive way of pumping more blood to an area to help with healing. However, we're starting to go down a slippery slope, because that inflammation is a fire and that fire starts to burn the house down.

—Dr. Darren Weissman

• •

Inflammation is an immune system response to either repair damaged tissue or remove harmful stimuli from the body. This self-healing mechanism might be temporarily uncomfortable and include redness, swelling, pain, or itching. Chronic inflammation, however, indicates a systemic imbalance that the body cannot correct on its own. It is overwhelmed, and we need to assist it in self-correcting.

As with everything in life, too much of a good thing can become a bad thing, which is why chronic inflammation can lead to diseases like rheumatoid arthritis, Crohn's, and many other autoimmune illnesses. The fact that negative emotions can cause inflammation to occur indicates that we must factor in our emotional health when we are healing. As Peter Crone points out, purely physical, conventional treatment may work for period of time, but if we don't address the mental and emotional factors as well, the disease condition has a good chance of coming back. We see this with cancer all the time. If one just bombards the cancer with chemo and radiation without making lifestyle changes or addressing the mental and emotional factors as well, the cancer may have a higher likelihood of returning.

Negative emotions not only have an inflammatory effect on the body but an energetic one as well. Modern science is beginning to prove what ancient wisdom has known for thousands of years: emotions are energy, and if we don't process them correctly, they can negatively impact the energetic systems of our body.

. . . .

Releasing Negative Emotions

In traditional medicine systems, [the theory is that] if the chi, the prana, or the life-force energy gets stuck anywhere from an emotional or spiritual level, and if that's not addressed, then over time that blockage will lead to a physical blockage. Now that's a theory. Western medicine hasn't proven that yet. But it is a theory that came up over and over again with the radical remission survivors and their healers that I interviewed. So, I think it's important to mention this idea that emotional blockages can lead to physical blockages. The idea, then, is to release them, and you can do that however you want to. Some people let it go in a Zumba class. Other people went to see a shaman and did soul retrieval. Some people did psychotherapy. Some people burned all the letters from their ex-husbands. It really is whatever's going to allow you to let go of that anger, to let go of that resentment or that grief or that trauma—especially trauma—which can often be locked away inside your brain in the subconscious part.

—**Kelly Turner, PhD**

When I was running a mind and body clinic, we kept coming back to regrets and resentment. I would interview people after our ten-week program, a program based on meditation, mindfulness, forgiveness, gratitude, and using the imagination, and what I would find is that some people just didn't heal. Almost always, the people that didn't heal were hanging on to regret or a resentment that kept them stuck.

—**Joan Borysenko, PhD**

There are so many different kinds of therapies available to help you release stuck energy and heal emotional trauma. Reiki, tapping or emotional freedom technique (EFT), neurolinguistic programming, eye movement desensitization and reprocessing (EMDR), acupuncture, qigong, breathwork, hypnotherapy, craniosacral, sacred plant medicine, chiropractic, sound baths or sound healing, PSYCH-K, theta healing, chakra healing, healing touch, float therapy, haptotherapy, and reflexology are some of the modalities that have been used successfully to help let go of obstacles and create space for healing. The theory that emotional blockages become physical blockages would also explain why forgiveness and letting go were mentioned by all of the experts as a necessary step when it comes to healing.

· ·

The Power of Forgiveness

Every authentic spiritual path has some mention or some teaching around forgiveness. I always say that all forgiveness is self-forgiveness because with the resentment, unforgiveness, or rancor I may hold towards another, all of those thoughts are happening within me. Even if someone did me wrong, I still have those thoughts, and those thoughts are affecting me; they're affecting my body temple, they're affecting my blood chemistry, they're affecting everything. So, when I begin to forgive the so-called other person, I'm releasing rancor, resentment, animosity. I'm releasing all that unforgiveness so that I'm actually forgiving myself. Now, it doesn't necessarily let the other person off the hook for whatever they did or didn't do or should've done or should not have done; it has nothing to do with them. It has everything to do with me.

—**Dr. Michael B. Beckwith**

Forgiveness, when it comes to emotions, is the greatest access to letting go. The hatred you have of a parent, the judgment you have of a coworker, the wrong-making you have towards your spouse—just let go of that inner judgment, blame, and basically a victim mind-set. If you can let go of that and recognize that life is actually working for you not against you, then you're going to generate healing.

—**Peter Crone**

. . . .

Who do you need to forgive? What do you need to forgive in yourself? What regret or resentment can you let go of today?

"Forgiveness liberates the soul. It removes fear.
That is why it is such a powerful weapon."

—Nelson Mandela

Once you have cleared your body of negative emotions, it's time to build up your store of positive emotions. While unprocessed, negative emotions can accumulate and cause inflammation and stress, positive emotions have the opposite effect—they can work to change your body's energetic state into one of healing.

When I saw the movie *The Secret*, the two stories that stuck with me the most were the woman who healed herself from late-stage breast cancer in three months by watching funny movies and the story of Norman Cousins who healed himself from ankylosing spondylitis. Cousins realized that his intense pain would disappear when he was laughing and decided to watch funny movies and television shows all day to ease the pain. "I made the joyous discovery that ten minutes of genuine belly laughter had an anesthetic effect and would give me at least two hours of pain-free sleep," he said. Eventually, with laughter therapy and IVs of high doses of vitamin C, Cousins completely healed. Maybe laughter *is* the best medicine after all!

"Humor can obliterate fear. You can't be afraid
when you're laughing, period."
—Bernie Siegel, MD

Kelly Turner told me about a study in which cancer patients were shown stand-up comedy videos while going through chemotherapy (another group was not shown the videos). Within four hours, the immune counts of the people who watched the comedy were significantly higher than the other group. "The result was almost instantaneous!" Kelly said. "Those people also had fewer side effects and they were able to bounce back better from the chemo."

Kelly admitted that it's not always easy to feel positive, especially when dealing with a potentially fatal illness. "The one thing that radical remission survivors really wanted me to come back to the world and shout out with a megaphone is that you don't have to feel happy all the time," she told me. "You don't have to worry that if you're not happy all the time, you're going to hurt your immune system or help your cancer stay. That's just a vicious cycle of self-blame, which certainly won't help your immune system."

Instead, using positive emotions to heal is sort of like exercising. You just need to do a little bit every day to reap the benefits. Kelly went on to explain: "I met people who said they were in deep fear for months, but they made it a point to distract themselves from that fear for at least five minutes a day—with a phone call to a friend or a cuddle session with their cat or by watching a funny movie. If you can just stop that negative circuitry for five minutes, you are allowing your immune system a chance to reset itself and start working. And that's what's important."

. . . .

The Biochemistry of LOVE

When a person is in an environment where they feel love—even when a person is thinking about that environment, thinking about a time when someone showed them love or affection or when they felt close to someone, it could even be an animal like a dog, cat, or horse, even—they produce oxytocin hormone in the brain, they produce it in their heart, and they produce it in their reproductive organs. Oxytocin delivers fantastic benefits to the heart. It changes the shape of blood vessels, and it sweeps out some of the precursors to heart disease and keeps the arteries healthy. It also plays a role in digestion, helping us to digest our food better.

So healing can be accelerated, so to speak, when we are thinking of love, compassion, gratitude, affection, kindness, and generosity of spirit. Love itself is the most wonderful, beautiful, healing thing, and

I love that science is now showing biologically what some of these effects actually are.

—David R. Hamilton, PhD

The chemistry of love—the interpretation of love is translated into some very interesting chemistry. Dopamine is a result of love, which is pleasure. Oxytocin results from love, which is bonding to the source of pleasure. When you're in love, vasopressin is a chemical that is released into the blood that makes you more attractive to your partner. Most importantly, when you're in love the brain releases growth hormone. When I am in love I'm actually enhancing the health and growth of myself.

When we talk about health in the body, we can talk about the body having two different directives: to be in growth or to be in protection. They are two different behaviors and are mutually exclusive. For example, when a stimulus offers growth, it's a stimulus that I want to move toward and take in, like love. I will move toward love with open arms and take it in. But in contrast, if the stimulus is negative and threatening I don't move toward the stimulus, I move away from the stimulus and I close myself down. What's the point? Growth moves toward the stimulus, protection moves away from the stimulus. You can't move forwards and backwards at the same time. You can't be open and closed at the same time. Growth and protection are mutually exclusive behaviors. Okay, so when I get a negative perception about my life like a diagnosis that is negative, I'm going to try to protect myself. I'm going to close down my system to ward off the problem.

Well, closing down the system is the opposite of growth, and that will actually accelerate illness and death. So fear leads to death. If you say you have no fear, I'll ask, "But do you have any love?" You ask, "What's the difference?" Well love opens you up to take things in. You can grow and heal. If you're not in stress and you're not in love where are you? You are in the middle. You're not growing and you're not protecting yourself. If you want to enhance your life, then you have to move from fear into love, protection into growth. The problem is not just eliminating stress but to eliminate it and replace it with something positive, loving, growth promoting.

—Bruce Lipton, PhD

• •

"Love is the greatest healing power I know."

—Louise Hay

The beauty of learning how to release negative emotions and increase positive emotions is that we can directly impact the health of our own bodies by using our thoughts. We can simply *think* about things that make us happy, think of a time we were in love, watch a funny or joy-invoking movie, and the thoughts and feelings have the power to release healing chemistry in our bodies. This is incredibly hopeful news.

An inspiring example of this is Joe Dispenza and his remarkable self-healing story.

Joe Dispenza's Story

In 1986, Joe Dispenza was competing in the cycling portion of a triathlon in Palm Springs, California. As he made an unexpected turn as directed by a police officer, a four-wheel-drive Bronco going about fifty-five miles per hour hit him from behind and catapulted him off his bicycle. Joe landed hard on his lower back and buttocks, and the compressive force compressed six vertebrae in his spine. One of his vertebrae was more than 60 percent collapsed and the neural arch where the spinal cord passes through had broken like a pretzel.

Joe had multiple compression fractures of his thoracic spine and upper lumbar spine, bone fragments on his spinal cord, and compression of the spinal cord because of the neural arch being fractured. At the hospital he got four opinions from four of the leading surgeons in Southern California, and the prognosis was that he would probably never walk again. He was also advised to try the Harrington Rod surgery—a radical procedure inserting long stainless-steel rods from the base of his neck to the base of his spine.

It was extremely difficult for him to weigh what he knew against what he didn't know, being a chiropractor himself. Even with all the X-rays, CAT scans, MRIs, and expert prognoses, Joe didn't want to have surgery. He couldn't imagine living on addictive medications or being in a wheelchair for the rest of his life. And as he decided to check out of the hospital, he had one thought: *the power that made the body heals the body.*

Joe believed that the same intelligence that gives us life has awareness, and it was paying attention to him. He decided to make contact with that intelligence and give it a plan for his own healing—a specific design for himself. He would surrender his plan to that greater intelligence because it would know how to heal much better than he could.

So, unable to do anything but lie there and think, Joe began reconstructing his spine in his mind, vertebra by vertebra. But Joe couldn't always get his mind to do what he wanted; he'd lose focus and think about living in a wheelchair and have to stop and start all over again. For six weeks Joe struggled—he felt frustrated, impatient, and angry. It would take three hours to get through the whole spine, closing his eyes and reconstructing every single vertebra in his mind.

"I was never satisfied really with the way it was, the way I did it," Joe said, "But I would just keep going. At the end of six weeks, I went through the whole entire process without losing my attention. Something clicked in that moment; I clicked. And I knew in that moment that something happened."

Soon, what took him three hours to complete now took him forty-five minutes. At the time, he didn't know it, but through the repetition and practice he was firing and wiring new circuits in his brain every single day. He was also improving his ability to pay attention—just like any skill, the more you practice it, the better you get at it. "I wasn't going anywhere. I wasn't doing anything. I was basically lying facedown and I had a lot of time on my hands," Joe remembered.

Joe started noticing significant changes in his body. His pain levels dropped and then diminished immediately; some of his neurological problems, such as numbness and tingling, began improving; and his motor functions started coming back. "The moment I correlated what I was doing inside of me with the effect that I was producing outside of me, I did it with more passion and more enthusiasm instead of dread and frustration," he said.

His thought process became fun and easy. "If I was ever able to walk again, what did I take for granted, like a sunset or a shower or sitting with my friends and enjoying a meal? I started selecting potentials in the quantum field that were no longer based on the worst-case scenario but really some future possibility."

Joe began to signal new genes in new ways, and his body changed dramatically. He was back on his feet in ten weeks and back training again at twelve weeks. He reports not having any pain in his body or his back. "I just made a deal with myself and the deal was with this intelligence: if I was ever able to walk again, I'd spend the rest of my life studying the mind-body connection and mind over matter—and pretty much that's what I've been doing since 1986."

Joe's remarkable healing story demonstrates for me how powerful the mind-body connection really is. It also shows that healing not only takes our full participation and focus but also commitment, dedication, patience, and enthusiasm.

If you are on a healing journey, where can you boost your focus and commitment? Can you dedicate ten minutes every day to visualize and imagine yourself healthy and once again doing the things you love doing?

Chapter 3 Takeaways

- Our beliefs begin in the subconscious mind, and we are often not even aware of them. If we can become aware of our limiting and negative subconscious beliefs, we can change the patterns that no longer serve us.

- The field of epigenetics shows us that we are no longer victims of our heredity. By changing our environment or our perception of our environment, we can actually influence our genetic activity.

- Our emotions have a direct impact on our physiology. Negative emotions can have an inflammatory effect on the body, and positive emotions can have a healing effect. Two of the nine key factors in radical remission are releasing suppressed emotions and increasing positive emotions.

- There is an actual positive chemistry of love that we can release in our own bodies, making it one of the greatest healing powers of all.

- Healing can happen spontaneously or can require time, commitment, dedication, focus, practice, and patience.

The Placebo Effect, Perception, and Belief

Whatever the mind of man can conceive and believe,
it can achieve.

—Napoleon Hill

Y ou may have heard of the *placebo effect*—a term coined
by Dr. Henry Beecher in a 1955 research paper, "The
Powerful Placebo"—you take a sugar pill thinking it's medicine, and you actually start to feel better. But how does this
really work? And how can we harness this Jedi mind trick to
improve our own capacity to heal, potentially without the
harmful side effects of drugs and medication?

I spoke with Joe Dispenza, who offered a helpful,
in-depth explanation of this powerful phenomenon. "People
can accept, believe, and surrender to the thought that they're
getting the actual substance or treatment and begin to program their autonomic nervous system to make their own
pharmacy of chemicals that matches the exact same chemical they think they're taking," he said.

Okay. But how is it that an inert substance causes a healing effect in the body? I wondered.

"The sugar pill, the inert substance, is not doing the healing, so it's *the thought* that's doing the healing," he said. "In depression studies, as much as 81 percent of the people that are given a placebo respond as well to the placebo as the people taking the antidepressant. So what's the significance of that? It means they're making their own pharmacy of antidepressants and their body, their nervous system, is the greatest pharmacist in the world."

As Joe explained to me, the placebo effect is based on three things: conditioning, expectation, and meaning. First, you give someone a real pill and it takes away their pain. Give them the same pill again, and again it takes away their pain. Then you give them a pill, but this time it's a sugar pill that looks just like the other pill, and because they've been conditioned by the repetition, their body begins to make the same chemicals that make them feel better.

The second thing that influences the placebo effect is one's expectation. You begin to expect something to occur from a medication or treatment, and the moment you select that potential, that possibility in your future, your body begins to physiologically change in preparation for the event. You can say to a person in a placebo study, "We're going to give you a drug," and if the doctor's enthusiastic, it actually works better to take away your pain. If the doctor is enthusiastic and the patient begins to expect their pain to go away, the patient begins to make their own morphine.

The third element of a placebo is assigning meaning. If you say, "Hey, you know, here's your receptors on the end of your nerve cells and serotonin has to be picked up in the synaptic space. This chemical keeps serotonin there so it'll remove depression." You're looking at the charts and you're assigning meaning to why you're taking this pill, so you'll produce a better result. The more you know about the way something works, the deeper its meaning for you.

. . . .

The Power and Potential of the Placebo Effect

I studied the placebo effect for almost a decade, and I'm fascinated by it. I think it's the most important thing for a healer or a doctor to understand, because it is side effect–free healing. The truth is that it operates on the belief in the potential of the treatment. Now, we are learning that everything from pain medication to antidepressants to surgeries actually rides the placebo effect or the belief, much of which is conditioned through our societal orientation to health and disease or the belief that this intervention is going to actually work. If we can engage in that mind-set shift in other ways, if we can fundamentally instill a belief that the body has this innate capacity to be well, and if we can align with that, then it's just a matter of weeks, sometimes days, before we feel completely different in our own skin. I think that is the most powerful element.

—**Kelly Brogan, MD**

I worked for one of the world's largest pharmaceutical companies developing drugs for cardiovascular disease and for cancer. What fascinated me even more than the science was what happened when we tested the drugs. In a typical trial you might have a group of a hundred people using a drug to prove that it works. You also have to give a hundred people a placebo for comparison purposes, called the control group. Out of the hundred people using the drug, seventy-five people may show improvement. But it's not uncommon to see anywhere from forty to seventy-five people also showing improvement on the placebo because they think they're getting the drug. I thought, "Whoa, that's amazing!" After seeing the same thing time and time again, I began focusing my work on the different aspects of the placebo effect. I wanted to educate people on the mind-body connection.

The placebo effect is extraordinarily powerful because it demonstrates that belief itself shifts biology. The brain is like a pharmacy, and if a person believes that they're going to have relief of pain, for example, their mind causes their brain to look through its pharmacy and ask, "Okay, of all my different chemical substances here in my brain, what will deliver the pain relief the patient is expecting?" It turns out there is a natural version of morphine called endogenous opiates that get released into the body. So the person gets a pain-killing effect because the brain already has what it needs to deliver what they're expecting to occur. That is such a powerful find because it shows that expectation, belief, and what you're thinking about can actually have all of these different biological effects in the body.

Conditioning is when a person's belief is amplified over a few days. For example, a person might be given morphine for pain for two or three days. Then on the fourth day, it's secretly swapped for a placebo, just salt water, but yet the person gets the same degree of relief—research shows their belief is stronger because it's been conditioned over those three days. Conditioning really strengthens and reinforces a belief. **If you can find a way of amplifying your belief and expectation, you can reach**

deeper into the body's systems to deliver more powerful results.

Years ago, one of my doctor friends told me that the entire time at medical school, he only got a half an hour lecture on the placebo effect. The lecture was only about the ethical consideration about prescribing a placebo, and nothing to do with the actual power of believing something, the power of hope, the power of love, and even the power of the way in which doctors communicate with their patients.

—**David R. Hamilton, PhD**

I would tell parents to get a bottle of vitamins and put labels on them: anti-nausea, pain pill, or hair-growing pills, and give them to your kids during chemotherapy. It's amazing the benefit, because the kids have faith in them. I call it deceiving people into health. I got criticized for giving false hope, but what the hell is false hope? That's an oxymoron. I always say, "People do win the lottery; it's possible." I try to teach people what the people who exceed expectations do. It's not unethical. It's true. You have potential. That's the word I love: *potential.*

—**Bernie Siegel, MD**

A few of the experts I spoke to recounted stories in which someone was given the wrong diagnosis and then started to demonstrate the symptoms of the disease they were told they had. This is called the *nocebo effect*, a term coined by Walter Kennedy in a 1961 volume of *Medical World* to describe the counterpart of the use of placebo. Since then the term has also been used by anthropologists to describe the negative effects of belief. In other words, if you're told you're going to die, and you believe that it's true, your body actually begins to fail. Joan Borysenko told me about a man who was told he had stage IV lung cancer and had six weeks to live. Sure enough, six weeks later he passed away. A couple weeks after that, the doctor reviewed his slides and discovered that he didn't have lung cancer at all. It had been a lethal mistake.

Dr. Bernie Siegel told me about a man he worked with who was told he was HIV positive. It was the 1980s and this man was gay. He quickly bought in to the belief that he was sick, because he was witnessing his friends and so many others in the media dying from AIDS. He started withering away and showing all the other symptoms of the disease. A month or so later, very close to dying, he received a call from his doctor who told him there had been a mix-up at the lab and he was HIV negative after all. He never should've been sick! His belief and expectation of what was going to happen to him caused him to experience that fate. With a new diagnosis and a corrected belief and expectation, his body healed and he was back to being healthy a couple of weeks later.

. . . .

When Negative Thinking Causes Harm

What are the consequences of negative thinking? It's as equally powerful in influencing your life as positive thinking, but it works in the opposite direction. While a placebo (positive thinking) can cure you of anything, a nocebo (negative belief) can actually cause any illness and can cause death just because you believe it.

—Bruce Lipton, PhD

The word *placebo* comes from the Latin that says, "I shall please." The word *nocebo* means, "I shall harm." The nocebo effect is when I believe this will make me worse, so it does. Some doctors unwittingly tap into the nocebo effect just by the use of their language. I think if I had a medical school program, I would be teaching medical students and doctors not only about the placebo effect but also about the power of language.

—David R. Hamilton, PhD

. . . .

When a doctor gives a negative prognosis based on a classic bell curve of statistics, not only are they quite possibly harming their patient by catapulting the patient toward an unfavorable outcome, but they are also taking away hope. Isn't it more unethical to take away someone's hope with a negative outlook than to speak the truth and point out positive potentials, possibilities, and examples of successful, spontaneous healings? Science has demonstrated over and over again that our beliefs and expectations have an effect on our biology. Science also has shown that a doctor's enthusiasm or belief in a treatment or their patient's recovery has an effect on the outcome, because the patient's belief is reliant on and tied to the doctor's belief.

The moral of these stories is to get a second and third opinion! And be very vigilant about the language and demeanor that you expect of your doctors. As Kelly Brogan pointed out in the first chapter, our medical model and insurance protocols are forcing doctors to pack a lot of patient appointments into one day, often allowing for only a ten-minute visit each. Don't be afraid to ask questions or inquire about other options. It's often awkward or uncomfortable to chat during an exam, but you can ask your doctor to speak afterward in his or her office (when you are fully clothed), or schedule a separate appointment to focus on the discussion.

If your doctor gets annoyed or doesn't make time for you, it's time to find another doctor. In addition to paying attention to the way your doctor communicates with you, seek out doctors who will take into account your diet, emotions, stress levels, and other lifestyle factors. Remember, you have chosen them to advise you, and you deserve someone who has your best interests at heart. I strongly believe that most doctors have the best intentions; however, we need to seek out ones who have created practices that support the time and care their patients deserve. If you need help asking the right questions, find support from people who have gone through a similar diagnosis. They can share their experiences, and any tips and advice that may help you gain clarity about your situation.

Do you feel comfortable asking your doctor questions? Do you like the way your doctor communicates diagnoses and treatment options with you? Do you feel rushed when trying to ask deeper questions about your condition? Does your doctor have a hopeful, positive attitude or a cynical, pessimistic outlook?

Seek Support

There are many support groups available online, and healthfinder.gov/FindServices/ is a good place to start; you can browse by health topic and organizations. Facebook is another place where you can find supportive groups of people going through the same health issues and learn about potential healing modalities, inspiring stories, and practitioners. If you are concerned about privacy, note that a "closed" Facebook group means only members can see the content. And always be wary of a group trying to sell you something or requesting donations—they aren't all bad, but it's good to take into account the driving motivation of an organization. Look for groups that simply facilitate connections between members to share information and encourage each other through difficult circumstances. It may be virtual, but oftentimes checking in with empathetic voices, people who truly understand the unique circumstances you're going through, can be the boost you need to continue on your healing journey.

Sometimes, especially in the case of a cancer diagnosis, a doctor might rush you into conventional treatment with the honest intention of thinking that is the best option for you. Remember that cancers do not develop overnight. Take a few days to think about it. Get quiet, breathe, and try to calm the storm of fearful thoughts churning in your mind. Create space so you can listen to your intuition, do your research, and get a second opinion. At the very least you will then have confidence that you are making the best decision for you when you take that step forward.

The experts in *Heal* all agree that you should seek the best medical advice you can find, and receive your proper diagnosis but make your own prognosis. Don't let anyone tell you what you are capable of. Do your own research, find positive examples of healing, and guard your hope!

"Though no one can go back and make a brand-new start, anyone can start from now and make a brand-new ending."

—Carl Bard

. . . .

Believe Your Diagnosis, Make Your Own Prognosis

We give too much authority to someone in a white coat. I remember one time someone came in and they were crying because they had received a tremendous diagnosis and prognosis and the doctor said this and that. I said, "I'll be right back," and I went out and I got a white coat and put my name tag on it, which said Dr. Michael Beckwith. I went back in and said, "I'm Dr. Michael Beckwith, and I want you to know that your life is about to get better. You had a tremendous wake-up call and you're about to break that cycle of bad habits and you're going to watch your body change." Then I got a prescription tablet and I said, "Every day, this is what I want you to say to yourself, this is what I want you to eat. Come see me in thirty days and tell me how you feel."

The patient went from crying to laughing because she realized that she had given her power away. It doesn't mean you don't go to a doctor or follow good medical advice. But if you give yourself over to an external authority figure, you basically become a victim twice—a victim to the condition and the diagnosis and a victim to an authority figure telling you about what's going to happen in your life.

—Dr. Michael B. Beckwith

Okay, so believe the diagnosis—now you can do something about it—but don't believe the prognosis. A prognosis is when somebody says something like, "You have three months to live" or "Sixty percent of people die in six months"; it's like telling what the temperature is now by only knowing the average temperature for the year. If you're from New York City and the average temperature is 75 degrees, it doesn't tell you what the temperature is right now. There's no correlation. Nobody can predict your prognosis, so why not choose the best prognosis you have? Secondly, recognize the fact that only 5 percent of disease-related gene mutations are fully penetrant with our current stage of knowledge, which means in 95 percent of the cases there is something to do that could change the outcome of your disease.

—Deepak Chopra, MD

Statistics are impersonal, and you are a person. No one knows what you're capable of or where you're going to go. If someone says, "There's less than a 1 percent chance of recovering from the kind of cancer you

have," well then, someone has to be that 1 percent—
and why couldn't it be you? With the people that I have
studied, that was their reaction. They were all told
they had three months to live, and they all said, "Well,
if there's a less than 1 percent chance, then I'm going
to be that 1 percent, and I'm going to come back in a
year and tell you how wrong you were." And I love that
defiance, because it means they're willing to change
anything and everything to try to get well. They're not
all healing in exactly the same way. But they're willing
to go wherever it takes and to look at the dark parts of
their past, to look at their not-so-stellar diet, or to look
at their not-so-stellar relationships. They are willing
to look at whatever it is that's keeping their immune
system from working as optimally as it can. If they're
willing to go there, they can get there.

—Kelly Turner, PhD

I can't tell you how many people in our work were
given the voodoo curse that they had six months or
three months to live. They were told to get their papers
in order, their affairs in order, because they won't live.
Those people didn't accept, believe, and surrender to
those thoughts without any analysis, programming
their autonomic nervous system into that destiny.
They said, "Wait a second, I think I can make a change

here." And some of them either don't have the disease anymore or they're still living two years later and still making their way.

I think that it's important for people to take a certain amount of their power back. We're in an age of information, and in an age of information ignorance is a choice. Twenty-five, thirty years ago, you went to the doctor and she told you you had a certain condition, and she said, "This is the procedure that you're going to need." Most people just signed on the dotted line and said, "Okay, I'll get the procedure." Fast-forward to today and someone's given a diagnosis. The doctor tells them what their treatment options are, and they go home and get on the Internet and research that condition for hours, looking at conventional and non-conventional treatments and modalities. They walk back into the doctor's office and say, "Hey, I have this idea. I want to try this therapy" or "I want to try this," and the doctor either says, "I don't know anything about that" or "I don't think that works." People are now looking at their doctors and saying, "Time to find a new doctor. I want to find somebody that's going to support me and the type of lifestyle that I want to live, and help see if I can make the change."

Now there's a caveat to this. We tell all of our students that they have to measure. In other words, this is not about denial; this is about information. Which means if your values are high or your scan shows this, let's go for three months, and let's see what you're able to do. At the end of the three months, we measure. If it's staying the same or getting better, we keep going and we may add one or two other things. If you're getting worse, then you have to take a little bit more of a radical procedure to help you make that specific type of change. So this isn't about negligence. This isn't about burying the information. This is about really seeing if you can produce some type of effect and measuring it and getting feedback.

It's important for people to understand when they're given a diagnosis not to fall prey to the prognosis without actually considering that there're other options, without actually realizing they may have to do something differently, that they may have to make new choices, that they are going to have to get beyond certain emotions and overcome their limited thinking. If they can understand that, if they're able to do that, more possibilities open up as a result of their own personal changes; that's when you start to see all kinds of magical things start to appear in a person's life.

—**Dr. Joe Dispenza**

Miracle Mile

For centuries it was believed impossible for any man to run a mile under four minutes. After finishing fourth at the 1952 Olympics, Britain's Roger Bannister set his mind to becoming the first man to run a sub-four-minute mile. Two years later, on May 6, 1954, the twenty-five-year-old medical student ran the mile in 3 minutes and 59.4 seconds—it was called the "miracle mile."

While that is an extraordinary feat in and of itself, my favorite part of the story is that just forty-six days later, Australian John Landy beat Bannister's time and set a new record for the mile. Soon after, other runners started running the mile in under four minutes. Roger shattered a paradigm of belief and made it possible for others to believe they could do it too—and they did! It was an extraordinary testament to the power of the human body and spirit.

"I am brave! I am not afraid to face anyone on the track. I believe this is not a dream. It is my reality."

—Roger Bannister

How could you channel Roger Bannister's drive in your life? What are some areas of your life that feel impossible to change? How could you shatter that paradigm? What would it take to make the impossible a reality?

Medical professionals mean well. Most of them became doctors, nurses, caregivers, or chose the medical field because they believe in helping people and have a strong desire to save lives. But not all of them realize the power of their words or the effect of their attitude on a patient, and too many patients have left an appointment feeling less hopeful than when they arrived.

We need to take our power back and take more responsibility for our own health. Experts and specialists can help us diagnose a condition, but we should feel empowered to seek a second opinion, do our own research, and discover the things we can change, if they exist. More and more alternative therapies are becoming increasingly accessible and affordable, and there is a growing community of support as these treatments become mainstream. As Drs. Deepak Chopra and Joe Dispenza have shown us, in 95 percent of illnesses, there is something that can be changed, and the potential to heal does exist. Like so many people who defied what was thought possible and paved the way for new possibilities, you can do that in your life too. We live in a world of infinite possibility. Focus on the outcome you want, and you may be surprised to discover that you're closer than you think.

Chapter 4 Takeaways

- The placebo effect is based on three things: conditioning, expectation, and meaning. This phenomenon is extraordinarily powerful because it demonstrates that positive belief itself shifts biology. If you can find a way of amplifying your belief and expectation, you can reach deeper into the body's systems to deliver more powerful results.

- The nocebo effect is when a negative belief and lack of hope can actually cause illness, disease, or even death.

- Always seek a second and third opinion. Do the research and educate yourself. Find a doctor who will be your ally and make time to explore options with you.

- Seek support from people who have gone through a similar diagnosis, or join online forums designed to help share information with those who are also suffering from similar conditions.

- Seek a diagnosis from the best medical experts you have access to, but make your own prognosis. Consider all options and choices before simply accepting another's opinion about what's possible for you. Be brave, focus on the outcome you want, and trust in your ability to overcome and heal.

The Disease of Resistance

Accept—then act. Whatever the present moment
contains, accept it as if you had chosen it. Always
work with it, not against it.... This will miraculously
transform your whole life.

—**Eckhart Tolle**

The spiritual teachers I speak with often talk about staying in the present moment. Freedom, peace, grace, guidance, and enlightenment—these are all ultimately found when one is able to access and stay in the present moment. The experts in *Heal* agree that stress occurs when we relive regrets and resentments of the past or imagine worst-case scenarios of the future. Acceptance of where you are in the present moment is where freedom and healing begin.

One of the reasons I embarked on both writing and producing *Heal* was to shift the belief we have around certain diagnoses. Cancer is a diagnosis that will send most people into a downward spiral of terror because we automatically associate it with a death sentence. Degenerative and autoimmune illnesses such as ALS (amyotrophic lateral sclerosis), MS (multiple sclerosis), Lyme disease, and rheumatoid arthritis can also elicit a similar response.

On my journey I have heard accounts and testimonies of at least one person fully recovering from every stage of each disease listed above, including ALS. So it *is* possible to disrupt the paradigm of belief around these conditions. If it's possible, the more we focus our energy on possibility and potential, the more we can shift our beliefs away from fear around these diseases. Fear and stress only impede the immune system and accelerate the disease process. We need to disrupt the fear, stop resisting, and start telling a different story.

. . . .

Resistance Really Is Futile

You go out there in the world and everybody's got a shitload of problems. No, they don't. They have circumstances that they're resisting. Circumstances that their ego is saying shouldn't be that way. "They shouldn't talk to me like that." "That car shouldn't pull in front of me in traffic." "I shouldn't be sick." That's where the suffering lies. We're not in harmony with life and not accepting life. That's what will create a lack of ease, which is the precursor to disease, which then obviously gets manifested in our physiology. That's why I love the term *dis-ease*.

Let's say a doctor walks in and he says, "I'm sorry, I've got some bad news; your results came back, they're malignant, and you have cancer." Now that piece of information itself is just information. It doesn't actually change anything other than your perception, which will now create fear. That fear is fictitious, caused by your imagining the worst-case scenario. **The suffering is created by the story we tell ourselves about the information.**

The first step for any kind of healing and freedom is acceptance. Reality is reality. The ego mind would like it to be different, and that's where we suffer. Acceptance is where suddenly now you become in harmony with life. Then of course, you have choices as to what you want to do. In life, it's very simple: you do something about it or you don't. Most people do neither and they just resist it. Their resistance to the unwanted circumstance, their frustration about it, their anger about it, and their victim mind-set are all the emotions that are energetically precursors to it and will ultimately lead to its continuation.

—Peter Crone

We are not victims, we are the creators. If we put stress in our lives, then we manifest disease. If we remove stress from our lives, we can remove disease. The concept of spontaneous remission is real. People can have full-out cancer, be put on a death-watch, and then overnight get rid of the cancer. How? By changing their perception and beliefs about life, not changing the genetics.

—Bruce Lipton, PhD

. . . .

We need to accept reality, which may include a painful diagnosis. Resisting what is happening takes up valuable energy we need for healing. However, we don't need to accept our prognosis, or someone else's opinion about what might ultimately happen to us. In Kelly Turner's research, she interviewed a lot of people who were almost defiant of their terminal prognoses, saying, "No way will this beat me." That is not denying the diagnosis but rather a healthy resistance to the prognosis, which again, is not a reality until you buy into it. They accepted what was happening in their lives, and committed to change everything and anything needed to heal.

Think about pushing a boulder up a mountain, resisting gravity the whole way, and the incredible amount of energy that takes. Reality is the boulder, and the gravity that you are fighting is the natural intelligence that is trying to point you in the direction of your soul's evolution. When we are not well, we cannot afford to waste energy and suppress the immune system with fear and resistance. We must accept the present circumstance, trust that it brings a valuable message, take responsibility for our health, find our support team, and go through the difficult process of changing our lifestyle, removing stress, and addressing our emotions and core beliefs. This is true holistic healing. The challenge with this path is that it takes commitment and courage. Unfortunately, in today's society of convenience and instant gratification, we easily fall prey to the marketing of a quick fix.

Can you identify any areas of resistance in your life? What action can you take to accept your present circumstance? Can you change your perspective about the circumstance from one of resistance and victimhood to one of curiosity about the message, lesson, or gift this circumstance holds for you?

. . . .

Does a Quick Fix Really Fix?

We have the most money going into healthcare of any country in the world today, and we have some of the worst statistics in healthcare. The problem is this: the pharmaceutical industry is a corporate industry. What are corporations? They're systems where people invest money so they can make a profit.

—Bruce Lipton, PhD

Western medicine is a big business. I don't like to bring judgment, but to me, I think it is important that people understand it is a business. If the system of Western medicine were really dedicated to people's health, then pharmaceutical companies would be celebrating when drug sales dropped. Now I'm not in the building, but I don't think that's happening. The Western medicine system makes a lot of money because it's keeping people alive while managing symptoms, more than actually looking at the root cause of why someone has the imbalance in the first place.

—Peter Crone

In my examination of pharmaceutical products, in general, I began to notice a pattern. We are told that there's a problem, and the problem may not actually exist in the way that we're told that it does. Then, we're offered a product based on resolution of the fear inspired by awareness of this problem. We're offered a product that's going to solve the problem. But if you follow and dig into the literature, what you'll find is that the very product that's offered to solve the problem actually creates and perpetuates the problem it purports to resolve.

It's true for antidepressants and other psychiatric medications, which we now know can actually promote long-term experiences of depression. There's actually a term for it in the literature called *tardive dysphoria*. It's even true for acid-blocking medications, which actually induce a state of higher, more pathological acid production the moment you stop taking them. It's a pattern of the body's natural inclination to adapt, and when you introduce a chronic chemical in the form of a pharmaceutical product, the body does a very good job adapting to it and creating a new normal.

We have that and then we have to look at the efficacy. Do these meds actually work? Could those risks be worth it? That evidence is really even more concerning, because we have a body of evidence that suggests that these medications are no better than a placebo; a placebo, of course, which wouldn't incur those same risks.

I believe that it's every patient's right to know the fullest available picture of the risks, benefits, and alternatives to medications. Unfortunately doctors at large today are not in a position to have that conversation with patients because we are selectively exposed to literature that really supports the narrative of industry.

—**Kelly Brogan, MD**

I have nothing against pharmaceutical companies, because they've done an amazing job in helping people restore their health by helping them move back into chemical balance. The problem that I have is that I'm not certain that we're given the truth about how powerful we really are, because the moment that cat is out of the bag, you sell less drugs. So I question the efficacy of all drugs and what research papers are being published. Oftentimes, ones that don't produce substantial evidence that the drug works never ever make it into the scientific pool. Say there are thirty-eight particular papers that were written on a certain drug; you might only find eighteen or nineteen of those actually published. The ones that don't show any market results don't get published. So I think there's a transparency that's beginning to happen because people can become informed and they can find out for themselves.

—**Dr. Joe Dispenza**

. . . .

David Hamilton, an organic chemist who previously worked in the pharmaceutical industry, explained to me how drugs are made. Scientists at pharmaceutical companies take a plant from nature and may extract a hundred different compounds from the plant. They find that one or two or three of those compounds or substances works really well as an anti-inflammatory, for example. Then, the organic chemist takes that substance and, provided they keep the geometry the same, tests a bunch of different variations until finding the one variation that is a hundred times more potent than the original compound. That is what is eventually patented and made into a drug.

David explained that in nature, the hundred different compounds found in the plant all served a purpose. One or two delivered the benefit and the others abated collateral damage with the perfect mathematic ratios that are found in the natural world. Nature designed it that way in order to avoid any side effects. But the same is not always true with a chemical or synthetic version that comes in a pill. Side effects are common and often dangerous, especially when combined with other pills. Furthermore, the side effects can wreak more havoc on the body than the original problem the drug aimed to fix.

David's disillusionment with his role in creating drugs eventually led to his departure from the industry. "I started out as a young scientist because I just wanted to cure cancer. It turns out that most of my friends and colleagues in the pharmaceutical industry, all the scientists, also wanted to save lives," he told me. "It's only when you get higher up in the company that the goals begin to change."

This book is about awareness, not judgment. But I think it is extremely important to keep in mind that the pharmaceutical industry is a for-profit business, and the more people who are well and healthy, the less profit they make. It is also important to be aware that where there are massive amounts of money, there may be a lack of transparency to protect these same profits. This is reflected in the fact that some unfavorable studies don't ever get published.

That said, not all drugs are bad! We are so fortunate to have access to some incredible drugs and diagnostic technology. In acute situations like infection, advanced illness, or life-threatening injury, pain medication and certain drugs can stop the proverbial (or literal) bleeding and save lives. In an emergency situation, some medications and surgical interventions can get us to a stable, manageable place, where we can then support the body to heal naturally on its own.

But for the majority of chronic conditions, because of the multiple harmful side effects, pharmaceutical products may further knock us out of balance and require us to use more drugs to counter those effects. And lastly, consider this: According to a Johns Hopkins Study, iatrogenic illness—defined as illness or injury attributed to the action of a healthcare professional or a medical treatment—is the third leading cause of death in the United States, behind cancer and heart disease.[10] In order for us to have agency, take our healing power back, and make the best, most informed decisions, we must be aware of the whole picture.

> "Only by seeing the problems of our body and our world as a gift in very strange wrapping paper can we begin the evolutionary journey of awakening our spirit."
> **—Dr. Darren Weissman**

. . . .

Disease Is a Messenger and We Need to Listen

There is also the bigger question of what are you opting out of when you choose to manage your symptoms with pharmaceutical products. There's a story I really love which talks about a caterpillar that's in the chrysalis and it's struggling to get out of there. There's this little hole in the chrysalis, and a man nearby feels bad for the caterpillar because he sees it struggling to get out. So, he takes this pair of scissors and he snips the end of the chrysalis. The caterpillar turns into a butterfly that can never fly and dies, because it literally needs to go through the process of struggle and emergence in order to get the strength to fly. It physically needs to go through that to be able to manifest into a butterfly.

—Kelly Brogan, MD

People are going through an existential crisis. There is something in them trying to wake up. They go through that anxiety, and then someone gives them a pill to stop the anxiety. And that's not to say that sometimes we need to abate it so we can attain balance. But more often than not a person needs to go dead into that anxiety, into that restlessness, that pain, and see what's behind it.

Oftentimes, there's an old part of our identity that is falling apart. Something new is trying to emerge. We're afraid, so we want to cut it off with some kind of pill, some kind of pharmaceutical that's going to keep us numb, keep us cut off from ourself and block our creativity. So that crisis, that diagnosis, is the universe saying, "Psst, wake up." We don't want to anesthetize ourselves with our drug of choice. Sometimes that drug is fast food, busy-ness, cigarettes, alcohol, and sometimes it's pharmaceuticals. We want to stop, we want to look within ourselves, and we want to ask the right questions so that we can really change, transform, and become a greater version of ourselves.

—**Dr. Michael B. Beckwith**

There are times when Western medicine is the greatest blessing, but we often acquiesce to taking a pill for the sake of taking a pill because on one level we don't know any better. The Western world looks at pain, symptoms, or disease as a problem, but pain, symptoms, and disease of the body are a portal to our subconscious mind. Be open to looking at what you're going through in your life as a feedback not a fight, not a failure, not something to fix, but that it is actually a conversation. Now the challenge of this conversation of pain or disease is that it's a language that most people aren't versed in.

A pain in your shoulder might be from when you were eight and you were bullied. The digestive challenge that is going on in your gut might be from when you were three and a sibling was born and Mom was overwhelmed and you felt abandoned. The lower back pain might be when you were in utero in your mom's womb and she was feeling whatever she was feeling. Cells have memory and those memories, when triggered, cause us to react based upon the different aspects of the acupuncture meridian. So rather than just looking to destroy a symptom, make it go away or fight it, we must see it as a messenger. The symptom, pain, or disease is bringing you a message, and it's powerful and profound. Don't kill the messenger. Give the messenger, who's bringing the message through symptoms and stressors, acts of self-love. Give the messenger the five basics: proper hydration, good-quality food, great rest, exercise, and owning your power. That is the key for accessing your fullest potential for healing.

—Dr. Darren Weissman

When I interviewed radical remission survivors, I was also interviewing their alternative healers: a kahuna healer of Hawaii, the traditional Chinese medicine healers of China, and the Vedic practitioners and Ayurveda practitioners in India. What they all said is that this body is not just here to process food. Our physical body is also here to help us process emotions. So, for example, in traditional Chinese medicine, the lungs process grief, the liver processes anger—different organ systems are responsible for different emotion processing. The idea is that if you have a lot of grief, you might have problems with your lungs. The location of the cancer from a traditional Chinese medicine standpoint is often an indication of where the emotional work needs to happen. So thyroid cancer or throat cancer could be related to the fifth chakra, and the need for finding your voice and speaking out.

—Kelly Turner, PhD

. . . .

After interviewing the experts in this book, I am more convinced than ever that the human body is an intelligent system in which our biology is deeply connected to our mind, emotions, and consciousness. Our body is our greatest ally and is in constant communication with us, trying to support us in the evolution of our soul. In the ancient traditions, different emotions are associated with different organs, and different body parts are connected energetically to different organs through the acupuncture meridians. There is a code that many integrative doctors, shamans, Ayurvedic and Chinese medicine doctors, and healers are cracking, and it has proven beyond any shadow of a doubt that everything is connected and has meaning; we just need to learn how to speak the language of the body as the subconscious mind. What a fascinating and intelligent system!

Learn the Language of the Body

There are many different modalities that allow us to translate the language of the body and the subconscious mind. Applied kinesiology, or muscle testing, is one way to decipher the root cause of a symptom or condition. Muscle testing was developed in 1964 by a chiropractor named Dr. George Goodheart. He discovered that every muscle in the body is connected to different acupuncture meridians, and these energy pathways, as defined by traditional Chinese medicine, also connect to every organ and gland. We are literally a giant, intricate jigsaw puzzle. As with many alternative modalities there will always be skeptics, and muscle testing is a useful tool that hasn't yet been fully embraced by the scientific community. But I have met and worked with many holistic and integrative practitioners that have had great success in diagnosing root causes of illness, imbalance, or infection that failed to present with conventional testing. You can search for accredited practitioners through the International College of Applied Kinesiology's website (icak.com).

Darren Weissman has developed a system called the Lifeline Technique, which uses muscle testing as the means to access the unprocessed emotions and traumas still sitting in the subconscious mind and body. "Muscle testing is, at least what I found so far, the most effective way for knowing when fear has taken the wheel of your life, and through it, we can discover what is at the source of a so-called problem, disease state, or negative pattern," says Darren.

Darren explained to me that muscle testing is literally just a reflex, just as if you were to shine a light into the eye and the pupillary reflex would trigger, or you tap on the patellar tendon and the leg kicks. Muscle testing taps into that same system. You're either in an active state, moving toward something, or in a reactive, fear-based protective state, moving away or avoiding something. That's the way the nervous system works: Sympathetic is fight or flight, while parasympathetic is healing, regenerating, relaxing. Muscle testing is a very simple way for anyone to discover when they're being emotionally triggered by a past trauma that hasn't been processed, or when a substance weakens the body, or when an energy pathway or organ system is weakened or blocked. Once he discovers what's at the root of the dis-ease, Darren then has a unique technique to process the blocked emotion and move the stuck energy. He has seen people improve and heal from all kinds of conditions, including cancer, Parkinson's, bipolar disorder, depression, severe allergies, autoimmune illness, and more.

Quantum Reflex Analysis also uses applied kinesiology and the bio-energetic field of the body to diagnose nutritional deficiencies, weaknesses, and imbalances in the body. Theta healing and PSYCH-K are two other healing modalities that utilize muscle testing.

Hypnotherapy is another modality that can be used to translate and decipher the messages of the body. According to Stanford University's integrative medicine clinic, "Hypnosis is a normal state of aroused, attentive, and highly focused concentration—comparable to being so absorbed in a movie or novel that one loses awareness of his or her surroundings."[11] Hypnotherapy gets a patient beyond the rational mind to discover the emotional trauma at the root of an addictive behavior, a condition of the body, such as chronic pain or cancer, and mental health issues, such as PTSD (post-traumatic stress disorder) and depression. Once the therapist discovers what is at the root, they can guide the patient to reframe the incident and effectively reprogram their subconscious mind to a healthier state.

Hypnotherapy is so effective that women are choosing to utilize it in childbirth to reduce pain. MD Anderson Cancer Center in Houston is also having great success with using hypnosis during surgery in order to reduce the use of general anesthesia. The numerous studies demonstrating the power of hypnosis to reduce pain, anxiety, and addictions are not only promising but also further indicate the tremendous connection between our subconscious mind and our physical health.

> "Life will give you whatever experience is most helpful for the evolution of your consciousness."
> **—Eckhart Tolle**

. . . .

A Health Crisis Can Be Our Greatest Gift

What I've learned is that if you talk to someone who's had cancer, they will tell you that the greatest gift they were ever given was the diagnosis of cancer, because it changed everything about them, and it gave them the opportunity to actually let go, trust, and believe. It teaches you so much.

> **—Rob Wergin**

I remember when I first came back, even with the negative experiences in life, I would feel thankful that I was getting an opportunity to experience it. All of our experiences are gifts because we've chosen to come here and experience life. I now look back and see that even having my cancer was a gift, because it brought me to where I am today.

—**Anita Moorjani**

In hindsight, even the darkest parts of my life are all something that contributed to who I am today, and for that I'm grateful.

—**Peter Crone**

People grow through crisis. If you ask wise people how they grew, most tell you a story of having had a terrible illness or, God forbid, having lost a child or having gotten divorced. Whatever it is, it breaks the pattern. It breaks the matrix. Whatever the difficult thing is, the beauty of danger and opportunity is it shatters your life—all the stories you were telling yourself, and the way that you hold your reality together. It's like Joseph Campbell's hero's journey, which is the rite of passage behind almost every Hollywood movie— who you were dies so you can reconfigure at a whole new level. The physicist Ilya Prigogine won a Nobel Prize for his Law of Dissipative Structures. He said, "It's true at every level: As above, so below. From the molecules to the farthest reaches of the farthest universe, things break down so that they can reconfigure at a higher level."

—Joan Borysenko, PhD

. . . .

The Chinese word for "crisis" is made up of two characters: one that can be translated as "danger" and another that can be interpreted as "opportunity." I think this is such a beautiful representation of what we mean when we say that disease and crisis can be our greatest gift. Sometimes we wake up after a gentle nudge from the universe. Other times, as Dr. Beckwith taught me, we must be hit over the head by a cosmic two-by-four before it gets our attention. Either way, in order to grow into our greatest expression of ourselves, we must walk through a fire of spiritual and sometimes physical alchemy.

Elizabeth Craig's Story

Elizabeth Craig was always super health conscious—not only did she eat a mostly vegetarian, organic, and raw diet, but she also studied and practiced acupuncture and yoga. But her life wasn't without stress. In 2010 she got married, gave up her business and friends, and moved from her home in Florida to an apartment in California. Then, in 2011, her mother died suddenly of cancer and Elizabeth was stricken with grief. Her marriage and homelife took a steep downturn at about the same time, and she felt sad, lonely, resentful, and afraid. Elizabeth continued to do yoga and tried to stay positive, but her foundation was shaken. She frequently got headaches and felt nauseated, and finally recognized there might be something wrong.

"I went to a doctor three times over the course of a year, and each time he gave me a different test," she said. "But the answer was always, 'Oh, you're fine.' So, the third time, I told him I had a lot of pain near the bottom of my colon, at the junction of the rectum. He did a sigmoidoscopy and there it was."

At first, Elizabeth's doctors thought she had stage II or III cancer, but a PET scan showed that it had spread to a few places, including her liver. To her shock, she had stage IV anal cancer. Elizabeth had never heard of anyone surviving from stage IV so, terrified, she flew to Memorial Sloan Kettering Cancer Center in New York City for a second opinion. "Even after my mom passed away, it was so hard for me to believe that I had been diagnosed with cancer," she told me. "I thought that I had done everything right."

After the second opinion confirmed her diagnosis, Elizabeth felt rushed into chemo and radiation. She was told that the protocol was a minimum of two years of chemo, radiation, then surgery, and finally more chemo. The statistics on this particular cancer and stage were a 3 to 10 percent chance of survival. Given her background in acupuncture and lifelong dedication to natural medicine and healing, she felt drawn to juicing and holistic treatments. "My brother, a rocket scientist, said to me, 'Lizzie, you've been juicing your whole life; more juice isn't going to save you. You've got stage IV. You're not going to make it if you don't do the chemo.'" It still took Elizabeth another month and a half before she felt ready to start chemo.

In the meantime, Elizabeth decided she would do all the alternative therapies she could to support her healing process, and she would chronicle the journey in hope that maybe someone else would benefit from her experience. One of the first people she saw was a Quantum Reflex Analysis doctor. After some testing, this doctor discovered that a prior root canal had led to a lingering infection. (It turns out that a significant percentage of people diagnosed with cancer have had a root canal that was not properly cleaned before closing it up. The chronic, low-grade infection in the tooth cavity that is no longer getting any blood supply constantly taxes the immune system, which then allows cancer cell growth and proliferation in other parts of the body.) Elizabeth had the tooth removed and the infection cleaned, and then began a complete detox of her liver, gallbladder, and kidneys to rid her body of toxins. She also attended Agape International

Spiritual Center to gain inspiration and strength from the Dr. Michael B. Beckwith's sermons. "It seemed like every time I would walk into Agape, Beckwith would deliver exactly the message I needed to hear," Elizabeth recalled.

With a strengthened faith from Agape and the support of her friends and family (who had started a GoFundMe account to help pay for her mounting medical bills), Elizabeth finally felt ready to start chemotherapy treatment. One of the top oncologists she met with announced that there were five chemo protocols for her type and stage of cancer, and that they would try them each in order. He said, "If the first one doesn't work, we'll try the second, and so on, but . . . well, don't worry about that last one because you probably won't make it that far." (Um, scary!?) He then slid a bag of peanut M&Ms toward her and said, "Your job is to keep the weight on. They serve a great cheeseburger in the cafeteria too." Stunned, Elizabeth turned to the friend who'd accompanied her and gave her the hand signal that signified, "Check, please!" She went out to find a different oncologist. After interviewing three more oncologists at three different hospitals, she found one who supported a more holistic path forward.

Outside her new oncologist's office, she serendipitously ran into Dianne Porchia, a spiritual psychologist, who gave Elizabeth her card. "Originally, the primary purpose for calling Dianne was so that I could die not afraid—because

I was afraid to die, and everyone said my chances weren't looking good," she told me. "But instead, after a few sessions, I started to feel miracles." Her first session with Dianne was on the same day she received her first round of chemo via a pack that she would wear for four days—a tremendously daunting first step in her cancer treatment. Dianne coached Elizabeth through both her fear of chemo invading her body, and her belief that it was poison, saying, "This is medicine and it's going to heal you; it's good for you." She helped Elizabeth relate to it as targeted medicine, like little Pac-Man characters gobbling up the cancer cells while keeping all the healthy cells and tissues intact. Dianne essentially helped Elizabeth redefine her belief about chemo by assigning a new meaning to it, a new visual.

"Because he was my little chemo pack, I started calling him Chemo-sabe," Elizabeth recounted with a chuckle. "Dianne really helped me change my attitude and see him as medicine, not poison."

Elizabeth and Dianne worked together twice a week to release old behavior and thought patterns, and bring Elizabeth back from a state of internalized stress to an inner state of balance and well-being. Elizabeth was surprised to discover that despite her positive outlook and her generous personality, she had stuck negative energy and unprocessed trauma related to her childhood. Based on an experience in grade school, Dianne helped Elizabeth see that she had developed a belief about herself that she was pathetic. That belief went on to create and attract experiences and relationships in life that affirmed this subconscious belief of "I am pathetic." And because it was subconscious, she had no idea she felt that way, or that this disempowering belief system was dictating her life choices.

"I didn't know that I had such a detrimental mind-set. I never wanted to be a burden, so it was always easier for me to give love than to ask for it. I had to learn how to ask for help and to connect. To love and be loved. When you get diagnosed with cancer, everybody comes out of the woodwork to tell you how much they care about you, and that's beautiful. That was more healing than anything."

Over the next six weeks, Elizabeth went to see Anita Moorjani speak, and found overwhelming inspiration and hope. It was a pivotal experience. She began to believe she had a chance at beating the cancer. She read inspirational books like *Crazy Sexy Cancer*; *Peace, Love and Healing*; and *Radical Remission*, all of which bolstered her belief that healing was possible. She went to a healing circle called a Daré and to an Indian sweat lodge, where the shaman gave her a bowl of tobacco to take home, to cast all of her fear and negative thoughts into. All of those experiences repeated the same theme, that healing was possible if she could let go of the fear and the negative thoughts and emotions.

Near the end of the first round of chemo, Elizabeth felt especially weak so she called Dianne to cancel their scheduled session. Dianne decided to drive to Elizabeth's home, where she found Elizabeth curled up on the floor, shaking. Her temperature had spiked to 103.5 degrees, so they immediately rushed to the hospital. Nurses and doctors administered bags of antibiotics, one after another, and covered her with cold packs, but nothing was working. "I could hear my heartbeat," Elizabeth remembered, "and it was like water and air pulsing in my ears, really loudly. The fever kept going up, the nurses were scurrying around, and I wondered if this was the end. Twenty-four hours later, I woke up to find my brother standing on the other side of the glass walls with a laptop. He showed me a group prayer happening for me on Facebook with over a hundred people participating—I thought, wow, that is amazing. I could almost feel the loving prayer."

Elizabeth left the hospital and shortly thereafter completed her first round of chemo and radiation. One month after completion, she went back to her doctor to get a PET scan to see how well the treatment worked. Her fear was palpable. The oncologist sat her down and said, "Well, your scans came back all clear." *NO CANCER*. A cancer diagnosis that was thought to need aggressive treatment for at least two years—and had a 3 to 10 percent survival rate—had resolved in a matter of months.

"I just started crying and laughing at the same time," Elizabeth said. "And then the doctor said they must have misdiagnosed me."

While I find the suggestion of misdiagnosing stage IV cancer after putting a patient through aggressive treatment protocols absolutely ridiculous, the truth is that the doctor simply couldn't believe that stage IV cancer could be resolved so quickly, based on his education. Even during the treatment, Elizabeth should have lost all of her hair from the cocktail of chemo drugs she was taking. With one of the drugs it was likely, but with the combination of the two drugs, all her hair was definitely expected to fall out. But in the end Elizabeth still had almost two-thirds of her hair. This is another indication that the complementary treatments she was receiving simultaneous to the conventional treatments were helping to support her overall immune system. During treatment, when her doctor noticed the health of her hair and checked her blood work he asked, "Your numbers look good; what are you doing?" Elizabeth mentioned she'd been taking a lot of wheatgrass. When she asked the doctor if he believed in its efficacy, he simply said, "No, but whatever makes you feel better, keep doing."

On her third anniversary of being cancer-free, Elizabeth reflected on the fear that still exists within her. "My body wants to be healthy, but it's the head that keeps going back to fear. There were so many stories that people would share with me about their loved one having cancer, going into remission, and then two years later the cancer comes back and they die within a few months. Also, the tendency for a cancer survivor is to think that every time something is wrong with the body, or they feel a tinge of pain, the cancer is back. Because of that, there were many times I thought for sure the cancer was coming back. It's really hard to let go of that fear."

I asked Elizabeth about the most profound lesson she learned on her healing journey. She told me that the most powerful realization occurred toward the end of the chemo and radiation. She wasn't feeling well, and she asked her brother to bring her to the beach to lie in the sun and watch people enjoying life. "As I saw people playing volleyball, running, riding bikes, and laughing with their friends, I just wish I could've told each of them, 'You're so fortunate.' It occurred to me that this life is as beautiful or as terrible as you make it, and we have so much beauty and opportunity around us. I just wish I could let them all know what an amazing gift it is to be alive."

For Elizabeth, cancer turned out to be a blessing. She admits that it sounds odd, but for some reason she feels cancer is the most beautiful thing that ever happened to her. It gave her insight, gratitude, and a different outlook on life. "It taught me so many things," she told me. "It gave me a lot of love." As of this writing, she has been cancer-free for five years.

Chapter 5 Takeaways

- Acceptance of where you are in the present moment is where freedom and healing begin.
- The more we focus our energy on possibility and promise, the more we can shift our beliefs away from fear and the worst-case scenario.
- Resisting reality takes up valuable energy needed for healing. However painful our diagnosis, we can learn to accept and receive it as a current reality.
- Once we can accept what is, we can move forward and start making new, empowered choices.
- We are fortunate to have access to effective drugs and technologies in life-threatening emergencies. But for the majority of chronic conditions, pharmaceutical products may further knock us out of balance with harmful side effects and require us to use more drugs to counter those effects.
- The human body is an intelligent system, and we must learn to speak its language. Our body is our greatest ally and is in constant communication with us, trying to support us in the evolution of our soul.
- Sometimes a health crisis can actually serve as a wake-up call, a gift of sorts, to allow us to grow into the greatest expression of ourselves.

Food and Nature as Medicine

Let thy food be thy medicine,
and thy medicine be thy food.

—**Hippocrates**

Most all the ancient wisdom traditions believe that food is medicine and that nature holds the keys to health and healing. Even Hippocrates, the father of modern medicine, recognized the healing power of foods in his famous quote above. But what are the right foods to eat? What is the best diet for optimal health? Is meat bad or good? Are whole grains good for you or are they inflammatory? Is fruit good for you or does the sugar it contains lead to weight gain and health problems? The challenge lies in the overabundance of conflicting information out there.

When I took the yearlong course on holistic nutrition at the Institute for Integrative Nutrition (IIN), I studied every fad diet from the past four decades. One of the most valuable things I learned is that we are all biologically unique, based on culture, blood type, foods we ate while we were children, where we geographically reside, and so on. There is no one-size-fits-all diet because all of these factors contribute to how different foods affect each person. The term they used at IIN was *bio-individuality*, and I love that because we are complex superorganisms, and no one way of eating is the cure-all for every individual at every time. That said, whole foods in their natural state have tremendous nutritional and healing benefits.

Lifestyle medicine expert Dr. Mark Emerson explained how, through diet, many Americans are poisoning themselves into disease. "There's a blueprint to everything. A blueprint of how we're made, how the earth works, and so on. Anytime we shift away from the blueprint of nature and how we're designed, we get unfavorable consequences," he said.

He asserts that we're ingesting things we are just not designed for, such as genetically modified foods, chemical pesticides, processed foods, preservatives, refined sugar, and factory-farmed animal products, to name a few. All of these can kill off our microbiome, disrupt our hormones, and inflame our gut. Our body deals with these offending items as best it can, but there's going to come a point where chronic, repetitive bad behavior catches up with us. That's what he calls the tipping point. "Cancer doesn't happen overnight; it is a progressive, decade-oriented thing. It takes a while to get cardiovascular disease. It takes a while to develop type 2 diabetes." Dr. Emerson goes on to say, "It's just the sum of the parts of all the harmful things we are exposed to or doing to ourselves. It's a toxic environment that we're introducing to the inside of our bodies, and that's manifesting in different diseases."

Dr. Emerson recommends eating a whole-food, plant-based diet. "A whole-food, plant-based diet means eating unprocessed, predominantly plant-based food. That means vegetables and fruits and whole grains and legumes, essentially all the foods that are nutrient rich with phytonutrients and antioxidants. Eat food as grown; eat it how it comes out of the ground and how nature made it. Nature knew what she was doing when she put it together. Our bodies are designed to process these foods perfectly."

He concluded, "When we remove the offending items like the genetically modified 'Frankenfoods' and toxic chemicals and feed our bodies nutrient-rich, whole, plant-based foods that feed our microbiome and stimulate immunity, our body will heal way faster than it took to get to the disease. And that is the beauty of healing."

It's easier than ever to find affordable, healthy, organic foods at your local grocery store—most have at least offerings in the produce section, if not a separate aisle devoted to organics. Local farmers markets are often set up in community buildings, such as schools or churches, or outdoors in their parking lots. And CSA (community-supported agriculture) programs are popping up all over the country, whether through your employer, school, or online via your state's department of agriculture website. These programs directly connect you with a local farm so you can purchase fresh food as it's harvested. Eating local and organic produce will give you the best chance of consuming foods the way nature designed them.

Another expert on the healing power of foods is Anthony William, known as the Medical Medium. Anthony has a unique gift that he discovered at the age of four. While sitting at the dinner table with his family, he heard a voice outside of his ear, as if someone were sitting next to him. The voice told him to go up to his grandmother, put his hand on her chest, and say the words, "Grandma has lung cancer." Needless to say, it freaked everyone out! Soon after, his grandmother went to the doctor, who confirmed she did indeed have lung cancer.

Ever since that day, Anthony has communicated with this voice, who identified itself as the Spirit of Compassion. He uses this ability to help people find answers to their health problems when conventional and alternative medicine come up short. When I asked him how he handles his skeptics, he replied: "It's really not an issue, because I don't really run into many skeptics, to tell you the truth. I'm sure there are plenty of them out there, but when you want to help people and people are suffering and they've got chronic illness and the answers aren't out there, it's not about the skeptics. It's about the person getting better and the person healing. It's about what they need. That's the focus."

Anthony has become a resource for millions of people dealing with autoimmune disorders and mystery illnesses and symptoms. When conventional medical tests come back inconclusive, Anthony has been able to use his unconventional diagnostic method of hearing from the Spirit to find the root cause of people's conditions and then provide the steps that can bring healing. He talked to me about the autoimmune epidemic that is happening all over the world.

. . . .

Your Body Is Your Best Friend

Labeling an illness or condition or set of symptoms as *autoimmune* is tragic. Now it's not the doctor's fault, so we can't blame them. It's really not much to do with the doctors. It's a theory that is now taken as law when it's always been just that: a theory. When we say something's autoimmune, what we're saying is the body is attacking itself. Imagine you just went to the doctor's office and you were told you have Hashimoto's thyroiditis and you looked it up or the doctor said, "That's an autoimmune condition. It means your body is attacking your thyroid." If it were me, I'd be in the car driving home, pretty upset. I would lose trust in my own body and believe that my body was turning on itself.

The reason we call it autoimmune is because we don't know the cause of the symptoms or the disease or illness that's occurring. Look at psoriasis and eczema: cause unknown. Multiple sclerosis: cause unknown. Fibromyalgia: cause unknown. Rheumatoid arthritis: cause unknown. How is it possible to actually tell some-one it's autoimmune and that their body's attacking itself, when the cause is unknown? What's happening is there is a toxin and/or a pathogen that is causing the symptoms, and the body is trying to protect you from it. There's something in us that's causing inflammation, and medical research and science doesn't know what it is so they just blame it on the person's body.

The truth is, the body never attacks itself, and the body loves itself unconditionally. It's working for you all the time, no matter what, and it's your best friend. There's another very real reason you are suffering, and that's what I am here to share.

—**Anthony William**

. . . .

Even though Anthony has a slightly different perspective on what causes illness from the other experts in this book, he does acknowledge that there is often an emotional and psychological component to health issues. I believe the theories aren't mutually exclusive. While it's a fact that pathogens and toxins cause disease, I have also come to believe that unprocessed emotions, chronic stress, and trauma can compromise our natural defenses against these invaders, and make us more susceptible to outside pathogens and toxins.

Anthony William's Healing Tips

One of the pathogens Anthony William claims is causing many autoimmune and mystery illnesses is Epstein-Barr virus. He shares that Epstein-Barr, in its various stages, is at the root of Hashimoto's thyroiditis, multiple sclerosis, chronic fatigue syndrome, vertigo, eczema, and more. He also shared that heavy metal toxicity can cause or contribute to many illnesses, from autism to migraines and much more. While he recommends working with a functional or integrative medicine doctor on an antiviral protocol for some of the more serious diagnoses, he shared some of the foods, herbs, and supplements you can use or avoid to effectively get rid of these viruses and heavy metals:

Epstein-Barr is a hungry virus, so I recommend eliminating the foods that feed it specifically: eggs, dairy, corn, and canola oil are among the top culprits. Pork is also important to remove. You may also have to eliminate wheat and gluten. People commonly think gluten is inflammatory, but what's really going on is the gluten is feeding the virus, which is then causing the inflammation. Epstein-Barr also feeds off of adrenaline, so reducing your stress levels will help with starving the virus.

Don't be afraid of fruit! The sugar in fruit is not like refined and processed sugars. It's a critical form of sugar that we need to thrive. Fruit contains antioxidants and phytochemicals necessary for our longevity and vitality. Frozen wild blueberries are the most healing fruit on the planet and are far superior to larger cultivated blueberries. They pull heavy metals out of the brain and aid in the recovery from neurological problems.

When it comes to people that have digestive issues, bloating, inflammation in the gut, inflammation in the intestinal tract with colitis, Crohn's disease, and so on, they need straight celery juice. Drinking sixteen ounces of celery juice on an empty stomach can improve your gut health better than anything, which is one of the reasons I have been recommending straight celery juice for decades.

In addition to your diet, certain supplements, herbs, and minerals can be essential in strengthening your body's natural defenses. Like many people, you may have a severe zinc deficiency. Without enough zinc in your body, you can't fend off pathogens like viruses and bacteria. Also, if you're dealing with chronic illness, you'll need to get the right type of vitamin B_{12} supplement—a blend of adenosylcobalamin and methylcobalamin. I've been able to get doctors and practitioners to help their patients heal by telling them it's the combination of adenosylcobalamin and methylcobalamin B_{12} in the right proportion that supports the nervous system. It starts moving people out of MS and many other different illnesses.

Two other popular eating programs for healing are intermittent fasting and the keto diet. According to Dr. Joseph Mercola's website: "A ketogenic diet is a dietary approach that focuses on minimal carbohydrates, moderate amounts of protein, and high healthy fat consumption— the three keys to achieving nutritional ketosis . . . It is not only ideal for people who are suffering from chronic illness or obesity, but also for those who simply want to optimize their health."[12]

Finding the right diet for you will take some checking in with your body. Remember, your body is an intelligent system with built-in feedback mechanisms. The body always tells you what it needs, and our job is to tune in and pay attention to what it is trying to say. When investigating different ways of eating, tune in to what resonates with you and then try different protocols, paying close attention to how they make your body feel. Remember, there is no one-size-fits-all diet so always be sure to listen to your body and not the latest fad.

How does your body react to what you eat? Can you sense a pattern when certain foods have a positive or negative impact? Keeping a food journal is one way to start building awareness around actually "trusting your gut" and seeing how what you eat affects the way you feel physically (and emotionally).

"When diet is wrong, medicine is of no use.
When diet is right, medicine is of no need."
—Ayurvedic proverb

Peter Crone, a noted performance coach and thought leader known as the Mind Architect, was always interested in optimal vitality, even during high school and college. He came across Ayurvedic medicine (or Ayurveda) sixteen to seventeen years ago and thought to himself, *Finally someone knows what the hell they're talking about.*

One of his favorite parts of Ayurveda is something called *samprapti*, which is a Sanskrit name describing the evolution of disease. There are six stages to samprapti:

1. Accumulation
2. Aggravation
3. Spread
4. Localization
5. Manifestation
6. Diversification

Peter explained to me that the process starts with accumulating too much of what is called a *dosha*, or the quality of energy in your composition. The dosha could be fire, air, earth, or water in your system:

> Take fire as an example. Let's say a guy accumulates too much fire in his system, maybe because he eats a lot of spicy foods, drinks a little too much alcohol, and maintains a high stress level. He may have a symptom of a sour belch from time to time. Burping is no big deal, but it's a sign that there's too much heat in his system.
>
> The next stage is aggravation. Now, what was a sour belch becomes a little bit of heartburn. This may not seem like a huge problem today because we've got the solution—you just pop an antacid pill every day. In our society it's considered "normal" to have a little heartburn, right? But you're not actually dealing with the reason the imbalance occurred in the first place.

The next stage is spread. In this example, if the person is still putting too much heat into his system—spicy foods, alcohol, processed foods—the excess heat starts spreading. Perhaps now he has a little skin rash or irritation, or an upset stomach.

The fourth stage is localization. The excess heat that began with a small belch now finds a weak spot in the system where he's lost some integrity. Let's say the guy we're talking about was a football player in high school and maybe took one too many blows to the knee—that would be an ideal place for the excess heat to localize and find a home.

The fifth stage is manifestation. The heat manifests as disease over time and becomes arthritis.

And the sixth and final stage is diversification. So in this case, it actually alters the tissue system itself and becomes rheumatoid arthritis.

"When I first heard of this system, it was just so beautiful and so simple," Peter said. "Understanding those six stages, if you want to prevent disease, what do you prevent? Excess accumulation. You prevent buildup. Now, to me, the biggest buildup is in the mind. You build up trauma, you build up experience, and you build up doubt. *Why can't I do this? Why can't I get the job? Why can't I find the love of my life? Why can't I get in shape?* So you see that whole disease process applies to the physiology and the psychology. It occurs everywhere—psychologically, emotionally, materially. You go into most people's garages, there's an accumulation. They've got their $50,000 car outside and they've got a bunch of shit inside, right?"

Peter's gift is helping people let go of the buildup of suffering, judgment, and trauma in their minds. I love that he extends the accumulation described in Ayurveda's samprapti to our psyche and material possessions as well because it affirms what the other experts have found in their research: stuck negative emotion and unprocessed trauma block chi and life-force energy and impede healing. If you are on a healing journey, this is why it is most helpful not only to seek guidance with diet and exercise, to release the accumulated toxins in your system, but to also find ways to release any accumulated, unprocessed trauma and negative beliefs, and navigate through your present circumstances.

Just as Marie Kondo created a unique system for decluttering material items in her popular book *The Life-Changing Magic of Tidying Up*, we must find our own systems for clearing out our minds, bodies, and lives. Whether you hire a practitioner, read experts' books, or follow teachers online, there are a multitude of options to begin to heal past trauma, detox your diet and environment, reduce stress in your life, and develop spiritual practices to help you feel happier and more at peace.

"Even the material and emotional accumulation become an aggravation, a stagnation," Peter concluded. "It's a weight that you're carrying. It blocks space. When you block space, you block possibility. These things that people have—like guilt, anger, depression, or resentment—they're all based on holding on to something. It's the accumulation of trauma, accumulation of judgment. When you let go of whatever's accumulated in the system, you create space. Space, then, is the precursor to healing."

"The best of all medicines are resting and fasting."
—**Benjamin Franklin**

Fasting to Heal Faster

Speaking of creating space in the body, one of the things that kept fascinating me during my research is the concept of fasting. It is a part of every ancient medical and religious system. It is not only a means to reach certain spiritual states, but it also helps the body purge any illness. All animals fast instinctively when they are hurt or ill. Whether it's your dog, your cat, a lion, or a deer, when animals are sick they don't eat. They may eat some grasses or bitter herbs to help clean themselves out, but otherwise they find a safe place to rest while their body goes into self-healing mode. Kelly Turner likens fasting to turning on your oven's self-cleaning mode:

"I went to a fasting center in Thailand, where cancer patients go when it's their last hope. You might think that they are wasted away from the chemo, and ask, 'Why would they fast? Don't they need to eat?' But part of the problem is that their body can't absorb food anymore, because their intestinal tract has been so scorched [from chemo] that they actually need to fast in order to repair. They are finding that seven days of fasting can result in a year's worth of repair on the digestive tract. Researchers in Southern California are showing that if people do intermittent fasting while they're taking chemo, it will help them experience fewer side effects, and their immune systems will bounce back better."

According to Kelly, scientific research has shown that after three days of fasting, all of our major organ systems start self-cleaning. Your liver will dump all its old bile and regenerate fresh bile, and your heart will clean itself. The reason fasting works is that we spend so much energy every day digesting food. When we remove that task from the daily agenda, our body's natural intelligence immediately uses that freed-up energy to repair any damage to the tissues of the body and reset itself by dumping toxins in a big way.

Fasting Tip

Fasting is a great way to flush out whatever has accumulated in the body and the spirit. It all goes back to that innate mechanism within us to self-regulate and heal. Before you embark on a fast for the first time, consult your health practitioner and consider fasting under the supervision of a specialized center. The National Health Association offers a list of facilities that meet the professional standards of the International Association of Hygienic Physicians (www.healthscience.org/education/fasting/where-fast).

"Nature itself is the best physician."

—Hippocrates

Nature's Healing Gift

These days, it seems like the smarter our phones become, the more anxious and depressed we become. Florence Williams, author of *The Nature Fix*, contends that part of our angst stems from a lack of connection with nature. Florence states that the epidemics of obesity, depression, loneliness, anxiety, and vitamin D deficiency all stem from our "dislocation from nature." We are spending more and more time isolated indoors, in artificial lighting, staring at our screens, than connecting with and coming in contact with nature.

Indeed, nature has tremendous healing properties. A famous 1984 study by environmental psychologist Dr. Robert Ulrich looked at patients during their recovery from gallbladder surgery at a suburban Pennsylvania hospital. According to *Scientific American*, Dr. Ulrich and his team demonstrated in their research: "All other things being equal, patients with bedside windows looking out on leafy trees healed, on average, a day faster, needed significantly less pain medication and had fewer postsurgical complications than patients who instead saw a brick wall."[13]

While it is fascinating that just a view of nature can be healing, the actual contact with the great outdoors is even more remarkable. Earth's surface possesses a limitless amount of free electrons of a negative charge. Many studies have shown that when our bare feet come in contact with the earth's surface (also called grounding or earthing), we absorb a large amount of these antioxidant negative ions through the soles of our feet; these ions have the power to neutralize free radicals and thereby reduce chronic or acute inflammation.

Historically, our ancestors used to walk barefoot and sleep on the ground, receiving a constant bioelectric connection with the earth's healing negative charge. We have lost this crucial connection, which may be a contributing factor in the rise of inflammation disorders. Studies show that grounding for as little as twenty minutes a day can impart tremendous health benefits, which include improved sleep, faster wound healing, reduced stress, reduced blood pressure, reduced pain, and of course, reduced inflammation. So go ahead and kick off your shoes!

> "I believe that there is a subtle magnetism in Nature, which, if we unconsciously yield to it, will direct us aright."
> **—Henry David Thoreau**

The ground isn't the only healer in the great outdoors. Dr. Eva Selhub, a lecturer at Harvard Medical School and a clinical associate of Massachusetts General Hospital, says that trees release phytoncide compounds into the air, which have been shown to reduce stress hormones and anxiety, while improving blood pressure and immunity. A 2017 study published in the *International Journal of Environmental Research and Public Health* explored the effects of "forest bathing," or taking a walk outside while tuning in to nature. It concluded that the practice (also known as *shinrin-yoku*[14]) is linked to stress relief, lower anxiety, lower blood pressure, and more. Not only is it essential for our mental health to disconnect from our devices every day and spend some time connecting with nature, but it is beneficial for our biology as well.

Spending time in the mountains and at higher elevation brings certain healing benefits too. Gregg Braden told me: "In higher elevations our blood actually becomes more alkaline. There are a number of physiological factors that happen. The hemoglobins enlarge to carry the red blood cells, to carry more oxygen more efficiently, because there's less of it here [at higher elevation]. The alkalinity is a key factor, because we know when our bodies are alkaline they are less hospitable to opportunistic viruses, bacteria, colds, flus, and things like that."

It's also long been known that swimming or soaking in salt water or mineral-rich water (like hot springs) is good for us. The minerals in the water—such as magnesium, sodium, potassium, calcium, bromide, iodine, and sulfate—all get absorbed through your skin. These minerals have a detoxifying effect and have been known to speed up wound healing, reduce pain, increase circulation, reduce inflammation, stimulate lymphatic drainage, and alleviate skin disorders such as psoriasis and eczema.

> "The cure for anything is salt water:
> sweat, tears or the sea."
> **—Isak Dinesen**

While water itself, especially salt water, has tremendous physical health benefits, the mental and emotional benefits of being near or in bodies of water run just as deep. The air around bodies of water (as well as after a thunderstorm) is chock full of negative ions. These negative ions not only purify the air by attaching to allergens and pathogens, making them too heavy to stay airborne, but negative ions have also been shown to improve mood and depression. Wallace J. Nichols, a marine biologist, shares his extensive research about the transformational properties of water in his book, *Blue Mind*. Céline Cousteau writes in the book's foreword, "Our brains are hardwired to react positively to water . . . being near it can calm and connect us, increase innovation and insight, and even heal what's broken."[15]

"When we recognize the virtues, the talent,
the beauty of Mother Earth, something is born in
us, some kind of connection—love is born."
—Thich Nhat Hanh

What I love most about the healing powers of nature is that they are absolutely free and address the mind, body, and spirit all in one visit. Take advantage of the generosity of Mother Earth and soak up her powerful healing gifts as much as you can each day.

Eva Lee's Story

The following story is a great example of how everyone's healing journey is complex and unique, because no one's life and circumstances are the same. It is also a challenging reminder of how much courage, commitment, and sometimes cost it takes to adhere to a holistic path of healing.

As I was making the film *Heal*, I needed some documents notarized. Eva Lee, who works in my husband's office, is a notary public and brought me the contracts to sign. As she handed me the stack of papers, she quickly retracted her arm and apologized for the rash on her hand. Only then did I find out that for the past three years she'd been struggling with a mystery illness. I inquired about the condition in order to see if there was some way I could help. "In the beginning," she said, "I just thought it was a reaction or hive or dermatological thing. But then I started to get massive breakouts, boils that spread to my ears and my head. Then, about a year and a half ago, I woke up in the middle of the night and I couldn't move. The right side of my body was paralyzed. I thought I was having a stroke and I freaked out. Eventually I felt tingling, and the feeling came back to my body and I rolled out of bed."

Eva explained to me that she sought out a diagnosis from all sorts of specialists, including a dermatologist, a neurologist, and an allergist. She had a barrage of symptoms, but the tests kept coming back inconclusive, so they all just told her it was some sort of autoimmune disorder. They gave her literature and prescriptions for many different drugs, but she resisted taking them because the various side effects—from blindness to heart disease—were as frightening as her illness. She shared with me how incredibly frustrating it was that after she had seen some of the best specialists in Los Angeles and taken multiple blood tests, no one knew how to help her. Their only solution was to give her steroids to knock out the breakouts, without ever finding the root cause of the flare-ups. It was also exhausting and financially stressful, given all her other responsibilities as a busy, working mom. Eva expressed gratitude that her condition wasn't something worse, but the overall burden of it was getting the best of her.

A few days later Eva came and told me, "My little one, Quinn, always prays for my 'dots' to go away while dabbing my breakouts with holy water. After I told her that you were going to help me she said, 'See, God's going to help Mommy.'" It made both of us tear up.

The course I took at the Institute for Integrative Nutrition taught me that not only is diet the foundation of our health, but a lot of skin issues can stem from poor gut health or liver issues. I also knew that taking steroids for a long period of time would most likely throw off the balance and function of one's microbiome. As such, the first thing I did was connect Eva with clinical nutritionist and lifestyle medicine practitioner, Dr. Mark Emerson. He did a full blood panel on Eva and then put her on a whole-food, plant-based diet in order to reduce the inflammation in her gut and entire system. He was concerned that Eva might have leaky gut, which is at the root of many autoimmune disorders. Essentially, leaky gut syndrome is when the intestinal wall gets damaged—through bad diet, stress, or perhaps long-term medication use—and toxins and waste leak into the bloodstream.

After just eight weeks following his protocols, her inflammation markers dropped tremendously. Eva shared, "I haven't had joint pain since I started the nutrition program—and that was the biggest hurdle. Before changing my diet, I couldn't even go up and down the stairs to my bedroom; I had to sleep downstairs."

Both Eva and I were excited about the improvement. While I understood that diet was a big part of the healing process, I also knew about Eva's strained relationship with her mother, and I thought there might also be some related stress stemming from unresolved family issues. Eva was open and acknowledged that she might have to dig deeper underneath the surface in order to heal. "The physical aspect of it is forcing me to realize that maybe there's something more to it than just being sick physically," she said. "Past emotions that are maybe affecting me or things I've pretended didn't bother me." Patti Penn, a Reiki and EFT (emotional freedom technique) practitioner, was the next person I called.

In their session, Eva revealed some difficult, deep-seated truths about her childhood. Patti discovered that Eva's mother had dealt with mental health issues and regularly took Valium while Eva was growing up. On top of that, Eva's father left one day when Eva was around eleven. "He couldn't deal with her craziness either, so he just left and never came back," Eva told Patti with a nervous laugh. Not only had Eva felt abandoned, but she was forced to take care of things around the house at a very young age and become the mother to her mother, so to speak. She had to drive her mother to work when she was too young to drive, take care of the household chores, and care for her siblings. Patti started using the emotional freedom technique, tapping on Eva's various energy meridian points in order to move some of the stuck emotions and trauma from her system. The idea with EFT is that you bring into focus a negative emotion, traumatic memory, or an unresolved issue. With your attention on the issue, you or the practitioner tap five to seven times each on twelve of the body's meridian points. Tapping on these meridian points while concentrating on accepting and resolving the trauma or issue, and replacing it with a new, positive story, will activate your body's energy pathways and bring you back to balance again.

As Patti tapped on the various meridian points, she had Eva repeat her words out loud. Some of the phrases that Patti had Eva repeat as she was tapping sounded something like this:

Even though
it was a lot for her to take on,
she did it anyway.
I deeply and profoundly
love and accept that little girl.
It was a big burden,
but who else was going to do it?
I picked up all the slack
because I loved her,
and I wasn't going to abandon her.

The session with Patti helped Eva become aware of past emotional trauma that was still trapped in her body, as well as some belief and behaviors that had resulted from her painful childhood. She realized how, since childhood, she was always taking care of everyone else, while sometimes neglecting herself. She started building awareness that she was worthy of being loved as she now had people in her life that loved and supported her. She also realized she needed to take better care of herself in order to be there for her family. In other words, she needed to focus on her own health and well-being for a change so she could show up more powerfully for her loved ones moving forward. Eva reported feeling a cathartic release after her Reiki and EFT session with Patti, and they continued to work together to release old hurts and wounds over the next couple months.

I also took Eva to get a sound healing from Dr. Jeffrey Thompson, a neuroacoustic practitioner and chiropractor in Carlsbad, California. Dr. Thompson explained to us that every ancient culture throughout history has used some sort of sound healing ritual as part of their medicine practice, which goes back to the idea that ultimately everything is made up of vibrating energy. Dr. Thompson developed a therapy in which, using advanced technology, he is able to find the precise sound frequency that affects one's brain centers and causes their body to drop into the parasympathetic nervous system, or healing response. He explained to us that the autonomic nervous system is the master controller of the body, telling all the other systems what to do. The autonomic nervous system is either in the sympathetic response or the parasympathetic response. When you are in a state of stress, your body is in the sympathetic nervous system, or the fight-or-flight response. On the other hand we have the parasympathetic response, or the rest-and-repair mode, in which our bodies are able to heal.

Putting sensors on Eva's wrists, Dr. Thompson collected electrical information from her heart until he found the precise sound frequency that allowed her body to "push in the clutch," or drop into the parasympathetic nervous system. What Dr. Thompson discovered with his advanced medical monitoring equipment is that Eva was in a chronic state of stress. Even when she was relaxing with soothing music playing in her ears and the range of sound frequencies were passing through her body from Dr. Thompson's special bed, the sensors showed that she only very briefly dipped into the parasympathetic response. She would always immediately switch back over to the sympathetic nervous system. This clearly indicated that Eva needed to do some mental and emotional work to get her body out of chronic stress mode! Her body simply could not heal in that state, and what she needed now to stop the cycle of these terrible breakouts was some serious rest and repair. In order to switch off the stress, I suggested she try meditation, which was the tool that transformed my life when it came to stress.

But despite the many alternative therapies she tried, Eva continued to have breakouts. She approached me at the office one day. "I've been trying not to take the steroids, but all of a sudden, a breakout just exploded over the weekend. I have these massive boils all over my chest." She unwrapped her scarf to show me the large cauliflower-like boils, and my heart sank. "They're starting to merge together and get really huge and extremely painful and hot. I am constantly burning up, followed by the chills."

She left work early that day and ended up in the emergency room. The doctors immediately put her in isolation because they didn't know if it was contagious, viral, or infectious. She also had really bad abdominal pains. After she was let out of the hospital and I asked her what the doctors said, she replied, "They called all these specialists and ran all these tests and everything came back basically normal." I couldn't believe that after a trip to the emergency room and multiple biopsies and blood tests, Eva still had no answers.

In the hospital the doctors had given Eva heavy doses of steroids to knock out the breakout. Her dermatologist then offered her a prescription of dapsone, which is an antibiotic. Eva didn't realize the strength of the antibiotic until she went to the pharmacist and he questioned the combination, asking, "Do you know that this is an extremely heavy dose of antibiotic?"

Eva felt like she was forced to pick her poison. The long-term side effects of both prednisone (a steroid) and dapsone were beyond grim. Eva felt frustrated and confused that even after more tests and a scary visit to the ER, no one knew how to help her. Living in Los Angeles, she had visited almost a dozen of the best doctors in their fields, and nobody could figure out what was causing the breakouts.

"They give me drugs for all these different things without knowing exactly what's going on, but that's the process with Western medicine. It feels like, 'Let's just throw everything at it and see which one sticks the best.'"

I, too, was frustrated that the breakouts were still occurring even after all the positive changes Eva had made in her life. The only option she felt she had in order to keep up with all her life responsibilities was to take steroids, for immediate, albeit temporary, relief. I asked Eva whether she might explore a holistic path more seriously if alternative doctors were covered by her insurance.

"Definitely," she said. "The steroids are a $5 copayment, and they work immediately. If I could get access to supplements and some of these alternative treatments at those nominal costs, then I would probably utilize them much more often. I also just can't seem to dedicate myself; I don't know why. Maybe I'm just too emotionally stunted to open myself up to clearing more energy. There's just something that's blocking me, because it seems achievable, and in my condition I should be able to, but for some reason I can't."

It is important to note that when Eva worked with Patti Penn during the filming of *Heal*, it was the first time Eva had looked at her childhood trauma as having a possible effect on her health. Uncovering trauma is not easy, and it often takes time and a few different modalities to peel back all of the necessary layers and reveal the truth. For this reason everyone's healing journey is unique and complex. Some may spontaneously heal in a very short time like Anita Moorjani, and others may take years of commitment and work because uncovering old wounds can be just as painful as experiencing it for the first time. Also, since Eva was just beginning to become aware of what was offered beyond conventional medicine, it might take her some time to find solutions that she resonates with outside of the Western model.

As a society, we've been conditioned to believe that conventional doctors know best and that convenience is key. But it's important to remember, convenience often comes at a premium. What about the long-term effects that drugs like steroids have on the body? What about the daily stress of managing a chronic condition that just won't go away, or constant discouragement when top specialists continue to give you neither answers nor direction?

For Eva, and millions of people like her with a mystery illness, seeking help is an ongoing journey of exploring different modalities and trying different remedies. The holistic journey can become costly because few alternative therapies and treatments are covered by insurance. If you are paying out of pocket for an alternative treatment and the results aren't dramatic after the first appointment, you might be fearful of the financial risk of committing to something that may or may not work and abandon the therapy before it even has a chance. Eva's healing journey is yet another example that our traditional medical system is failing us and needs to evolve toward a more connected, holistic approach. A big challenge of this evolution is our current health insurance model and the need for more coverage of complementary and alternative treatments.

As of the writing of this book, Eva hasn't found a solution or experienced the kind of breakthrough revelation we had hoped for. When *Heal* was released on Netflix, Eva received hundreds of letters from all over the world, offering support and different recommendations from healers, doctors, and people who have gone through something similar. As she sifts through these loving suggestions, she continues to be incredibly resilient and has made some great strides on her healing path. She left her stressful job and is focusing on her health and family. She continues to adhere to a plant-based diet and still works with Patti Penn now and then. She also recently started working with a naturopath who intends to support her through the breakouts in a more holistic way, while exploring different possibilities of what's at the root of them.

As a friend, I will continue to support her in any way I can, and I pray she finds an answer soon. Her story is an inspiration to me of the courage needed to face past trauma and create space for healing that may involve big changes like ending toxic relationships, quitting a stressful job, or letting go of emotional attachments to certain beliefs and aspects of one's lifestyle. I remain positive that as more and more people like Eva become disillusioned by our current medical system and are aware of a need for more holistic care, the demand will dictate a new type of medicine.

Chapter 6 Takeaways

- Ancient wisdom traditions put forth that food is medicine and that nature holds the keys to health and healing. Eat food grown and raised naturally and organically, as much as possible.
- There is often an emotional and psychological component to health issues. Unprocessed emotions, chronic stress, and trauma can compromise our natural defenses against invaders, making us more susceptible to outside pathogens and toxins.
- According to Ayurveda, the six stages of the evolution of disease begin with accumulation. Not only accumulation of toxins in the system but accumulation of negativity in the mind. We must let go of trauma, judgment, and negative emotion in order to create space, which is the precursor to healing.
- Fasting is a great way to flush out whatever has accumulated in the body and spirit. If you decide to embark on a fast for the first time, consult your

health practitioner and consider fasting under the supervision of a specialized center.

- Nature has tremendous healing properties. Grounding, spending time in higher elevations, and soaking in mineral-rich springs or salt water can all have enormous physical health benefits and are relatively affordable and easy to access.

Tapping into the Intangible

Science is not only compatible with spirituality; it is a
profound source of spirituality.

—**Carl Sagan**

A s I mentioned in the previous chapter, many people are
discouraged from trying alternative or complementary health treatments because they are not covered by insurance and therefore appear more expensive. Remember, convenience also has its cost and often you either pay now or pay later. A solution might be less expensive in the short term, but often one will pay later with side effects or more imbalance when it comes to using quick fixes for chronic illness. Alternative healthcare can be a long-term approach, which may be financially stressful and frustrating, especially if concrete results take a longer time to achieve. The cost and effort of trying different modalities can add up before you find the therapy or practitioner

that works for you. That is why it is important to educate ourselves and understand how our bodies are intricately connected systems, run by a natural intelligence. When we can see the big picture, we have more patience, conviction, and trust in the journey. All this being said, our healthcare system is moving in the right direction, covering more and more treatment options with insurance—acupuncture, craniosacral therapy, hypnotherapy, and chiropractic, to name a few. And some of the most powerful tools cost absolutely nothing—we just need to tap into them with our hearts and minds.

Ancient practices such as yoga and meditation are two relatively cost-free ways to help bring our bodies back into balance. Science is now proving that these aren't just spiritual practices; they have real, quantifiable, beneficial physiological effects on the body as well. Yoga improves balance, endurance, flexibility, circulation, and strength, as well as greater body and breath awareness. Meditation relieves stress and anxiety, strengthens your immune system, and releases healing chemistry in the body.

I can say without a doubt that meditation has been a life changer for me. I actually crave it like a pregnant lady craves a pickle, because I get to release the tension that has built up in my mind. Or if I meditate in the morning, I can set a peaceful and joyous tone for the day. I learned Transcendental Meditation in 2007. Since then I have been given an advanced mantra, and I've learned primordial sound meditation at the Chopra Center in California.

I have a whole library of guided meditations on my phone. Meditation apps such as Headspace and Calm are popular choices that help beginning meditators. There are a slew of free, guided meditations on YouTube, but if you are serious about committing to a regular meditation practice, I would recommend taking an actual course with a qualified meditation teacher. When you understand the origin, science, and benefits of meditating, you will be much more likely to commit to a practice, which will lead to exponentially greater benefits.

Oftentimes, people believe that they are too busy or that their mind is so active or analytical that they could *never* learn to meditate. As the old Zen proverb goes, "You should sit in meditation for twenty minutes a day. Unless you are too busy, then you should sit for an hour." If my mind is still racing after a few minutes of closing my eyes and focusing on my breath or my mantra, I picture my thoughts as a wild stallion. I speak to the stallion and say, "Whoa boy, whoa, easy," and approach this wild, restless stallion with gentle words until he calms down and I am able to caress his head. Silly as it might sound, it helps to have tricks like this. The key is to not resist the thoughts that come into your awareness. Just breathe, let the thoughts come and go, and calmly return to your mantra or to the awareness of your breath.

After regular practice you will discover what works for you. And as for the excuse of being too busy? You will find that your brain operates much more efficiently with a regular meditation practice. So consider it an investment and stick with it. Like anything worth doing, it takes practice and consistency.

> "The thing about meditation is:
> You become more and more *you*."
>
> **—David Lynch**

. . . .

The Many Kinds of Meditation

Meditation has been around for thousands of years. The mind is yapping all the time, and it's generally telling us scary and limiting things. The mind is wonderful when you're using it as a tool; it's not so great when it's calling the shots. In the very first research on meditation, done by a mentor of mine, Dr. Herbert Benson said, "It shuts down the fight-or-flight response—the fear response—and it stimulates the parasympathetic nervous system of the body, and that's what heals." So at the very most basic level, meditation relieves stress.

—Joan Borysenko, PhD

You wake up in the morning and take a shower or a bath because you don't want to take yesterday's dirt with you out into the day. But if I wake up in the morning and I immediately go to television or radio or the computer or the newspaper, then I'm taking in all the stress of the world; so I might cleanse my body, but my mind is carrying so much stress. That's why meditating in the morning is as important as taking a bath. You are purifying your mind, purifying your consciousness.

—**Marianne Williamson**

There are many kinds of meditation. There are meditations that involve self-reflection, where you sit quietly and ask yourself, "Who am I?" There are forms of meditation that are self-questioning, which is when you question your beliefs. A third form of meditation is what these days is called mindfulness, which is a terrible word, because you're not using your mind when you're practicing awareness. The awareness of a thought is not a thought. And then there is what is called transcendence, which is usually using a technique like a mantra. The mantra is a sound that competes with your thoughts and ultimately takes you to a place where there is no thought and no mantra and you're just left with awareness. So, as we practice these techniques, we get in touch by and by with our core being or core consciousness, which in spiritual traditions is often called the soul.

—Deepak Chopra, MD

Your pituitary gland does amazing things when you are in meditation. It releases oxytocin, dopamine, relaxin, serotonin, and endorphins. Everything good that your body can make is released when you make this spiritual connection. There really is this internal process that we can flip on like a light switch. We can flip on these "juices of life," as they are called in yoga, if we just take a moment to connect. It doesn't have to be meditation or prayer—it could be going for a walk in nature—but your mind needs to quiet, your breathing needs to slow, and you want to feel that unshakable peace.

—Kelly Turner, PhD

We did an amazing study just a little ways back at one of our advanced workshops. We took one hundred twenty people and we wanted to measure their circulating cortisol levels and a chemical called immunoglobulin A, or IgA. We put them through four and a half days of training, and at the end, we measured to see if there were any epigenetic changes or chemical changes that took place by their internal work. We found that the majority of people's cortisol levels diminished, which means they were no longer in survival [mode] and they were no longer stressed. But the relevant thing that happened was that their IgA levels went from about fifty-one and a half to eighty-three, right to the ceiling of what's considered high, and some people were up in the hundreds. Now, IgA is the primary defense against bacteria and viruses. It's greater than any flu shot.

—**Dr. Joe Dispenza**

. . . .

The experts (and I) all agree that meditation, when done regularly, is one of the most powerful tools for physical and spiritual transformation. Meditation quiets the mind, drops us into our hearts, and releases the mental tension that has accumulated throughout our lives. One of Kelly Turner's nine key healing factors is "following your intuition," and a regular meditation practice will not only strengthen your intuition but it will also quiet the mental chatter around you, so you're able to hear your inner guidance. You can't follow your intuition if you can't distinguish it from the other voices in your head!

Imagination as Medicine

While quieting the mind can certainly help with healing, stress relief, and connecting with your intuition, consciously using the mind with visualization and imagination can also elicit a desired effect in the body, and even the world around us. Albert Einstein, one of the greatest scientific minds of our time, believed wholeheartedly in the power of the imagination.

> "Logic will take you from A to B.
> Imagination will take you everywhere."
> **—Albert Einstein**

Scientific studies have now shown that visualization—arguably a form of imagination—can be employed to help people recover and rehabilitate from all kinds of injuries and conditions, especially strokes, Parkinson's disease, and spinal cord injuries. In a study at Harvard University, researchers examined brain scans of a group of people playing just five notes on a piano for two hours a day, for five consecutive days. What they found is that the area of the brain connected to and responsible for the movement of fingers actually grew, like a muscle. When you learn or practice new motor skills, you exercise and change the part of the brain connected with those muscles, which is the phenomenon of neuroplasticity. The researchers also studied a group of people who didn't actually play the piano but imagined in their mind's eye that they were playing those same five notes, for two hours a day, for five consecutive days. The brain scans of that group were identical to the ones who actually played a real piano. The control group, who neither played nor imagined, showed no change in those areas of the brain.[16] Incredibly, this demonstrates that imagination is not just child's play. No wonder Einstein believed in its power.

The University of Washington Human Interface Lab developed research techniques involving virtual reality pain reduction. People in burn units put on virtual reality goggles and played a game called *SnowWorld* while their wounds were being cleaned. The study showed that in most cases, pain was reduced by more than half when the patients were playing in this imaginary, virtual world. The burn victims put on the goggles and immersed themselves in a beautiful and pleasant world of snow where they could earn points by throwing snowballs at penguins and snowmen. This is a promising use of technology to help enhance our imagination, making visualization easier, in order to help with healing or reduce pain while the body is healing.[17]

"No drug exists that can compete with the
healing power of the imagination and
the energy it produces."

—**Dr. Habib Sadeghi**

· ·

Imagine Illness to Wellness

What if I told you to do a simple exercise of imagi-nation? Close your eyes, see yourself go to your refrigerator, open it up, find a lemon, take the lemon out, put it on the cutting board, cut the thing in half, take a look at it, juices welling up, and stick out your tongue and lick it. Your salivary glands would go crazy, and yet it was all in your imagination. There's no question that what we imagine can affect our physiology.

—Joan Borysenko, PhD

For several years, I've been collecting stories, testimo-nies, and interviewing several hundred people who have used visualization as some part of their healing journey. Amazingly, what like 99 percent of them do is just take an internal picture of illness and convert it into an internal picture of wellness. That's it—illness to wellness. And they just do it over and over and over again. So, to give you a few examples of the strategy of illness to wellness: people who are getting chemotherapy imagine the chemo drugs as little piranha fish going and nibbling at the tumor. In their mind's eye, what they're seeing is the tumor getting smaller and smaller and smaller until it's gone. People in radiation therapy imagine the radiation as little bolts of lightning bombing chunks out of the tumor, but again the tumor is getting smaller and smaller and smaller until it's gone. Some people use the illness-to-wellness strategy by imagining a tumor as a snowball melting under a hot-water tap.

People with arthritis imagine taking fine sandpaper and smoothing the joint, polishing it, and then putting oil on it, making it nice and lubricated and smooth. People with cardiovascular disease close their eyes and imagine walking through their arteries with a steam cleaner and power washing their arteries. When all the crap comes off the walls, they sweep it up and put it in garbage bags and remove it from the body altogether. How you imagine what wellness and illness look like is entirely up to you. You can only do it right.

—**David R. Hamilton, PhD**

The Power of Setting Intentions

In yoga, meditation, and spiritual healing, there is a lot of talk about setting intentions. Joe Dispenza explained how intent really works:

> One of the privileges of being a human being is that we can make thought more real than anything else, and we do it all the time. The frontal lobe is the creative center and makes up about 40 percent of our entire brain. It's the place where we imagine, we speculate, we create, we intend, we have attention, and where we restrain emotional reactions. When we begin to think about a better way of being, a new possibility in our life, that forebrain begins to turn on. And because it has connections to all of the parts of the brain, like a symphony leader it begins to call up different networks of neurons—from knowledge we've gained in the past or experiences that we've had—and seamlessly pieces them together to create a vision. We call that intent.

He then went on to explain that when we begin to combine new networks of neurons firing in new sequences and new patterns and new combinations, we begin to change our mind, because mind is the brain in action. I set intentions all the time—I intend to succeed, to find love, to heal—and I'm often met with disappointment. Like many of you, I've created vision boards and have repeated many affirmations about my new intentions, but sometimes I keep running into a proverbial wall. So what is the hang-up? Joe Dispenza says:

> The problem is that most people don't combine that intention with an elevated emotion. The moment you begin to experience that future reality in the present moment, the end product of an experience is called a feeling or an emotion. With that feeling, the body begins to believe it's living in that future reality. The repetition of that cycle—visualization combined with an elevated emotion—over time begins to fire and wire new circuits in new ways to cause your brain to look like the experience has already occurred. The elevated emotion tends to signal the body in actively instructing and selecting new genes to make new proteins to prepare the body for the event.
>
> How we think, act, and feel is called our personality. And our personality creates our personal reality. As you begin to think about a new possibility and your brain begins to fire in new sequences, your brain is no longer a record of the past; it's

now in fact a map to the future. If you then begin to emotionally embrace your future before it's manifested—in other words, you're not waiting for your healing to feel wholeness, you're not waiting for your new relationship to feel love, and you're not waiting for your success to feel empowered—that's the old model of reality of cause and effect. **This new model is about causing an effect, which means you have to feel empowered in order to create your success. We have to feel love for ourselves and love for life in order for us to have love in our life. You have to feel whole in order for your healing to occur.**

Gregg Braden also shared a fascinating story about the power of combining an intention with an elevated emotion. In the early 1990s the high desert of northern New Mexico was in a severe drought, the worst in over a hundred years. Cattle were suffering, crops were dying, and it was really bad. A Native American friend of Gregg's, whom we'll call David to honor his privacy, called one day. He said, "Gregg, would you like to join me where our ancestors built this medicine wheel for prayer of rain today?" Gregg didn't think twice.

They hiked across acres of fragrant high desert sage, the kind that releases a beautiful scent when your knees brush up against the little leaves. They arrived at an ancient medicine wheel, and David sat down, unlaced his old work boots, and stepped into the center of this wheel with his naked feet.

He turned his back to Gregg, closed his eyes, and held his hands in a prayer mudra for a few seconds in silence. Then he turned and looked at Gregg and said, "I'm hungry, you want to go get a bite to eat?" Gregg was shocked—he had expected chanting, dancing, or some kind of ceremony. "I thought you were going to pray for rain," he told David.

David explained that if he prayed for rain, rain could never happen, because the moment we ask for something to happen, we have just acknowledged to the universe that it does not exist. We've affirmed the very thing that we're praying to change. Gregg asked, "Well if you didn't pray for rain, what did you do?" And David replied, "When I closed my eyes, I felt the feeling of what it feels like when it rains in our pueblo village. I smelled the smells of what it smells like when the rain rolls off the earthen walls of my pueblo home. I felt the feeling of my naked feet in the mud. The mud is there because there's been so much rain. And I gave thanks of gratitude and appreciation for the rain that has already happened."

They headed back to Taos, the nearest town, for lunch. By the time Gregg returned home, he saw something that hadn't been seen for a long time. Big black clouds came in over the Sangre de Cristo Mountains. By nightfall it started to rain, and it rained all night and all the next morning into afternoon. It rained so much the fields were flooded, the roads were flooded, and cattle were stranded. Gregg called David and said, "David, what in the world is happening? This is a mess! It's flooding everywhere." David was silent just for a moment and then said, "Gregg, that's the part of the prayer the ancestors could never figure out. They could bring the rain; they couldn't tell it how much rain to bring."

No one can say whether David's prayer created the rain. But to Gregg there was a high correlation between the time that prayer was offered and when the clouds came in— clouds that had not appeared for months in that localized geographic area. Gregg watched the weather reports and saw that the jet stream came across the west and just as it got to Wyoming it dipped down in Colorado and in New Mexico and made a little turn and came right back up, right over the place where the rain had happened. The weatherman stepped back and simply said, "Huh."

Is it possible that one man's heartfelt gratitude could have such an influence on our physical environment? And what does that say about our ability to influence our physical healing? It makes me look at prayer in a whole new way!

"The struggle ends when gratitude begins."
—**Neale Donald Walsch**

The Frequency of Gratitude

Gratitude is a powerful creative force and a great tool to help you move out of fear. This all sounds well and good, but getting into a state of gratitude when you are faced with something terrifying is easier said than done! I know that when I am sick or in pain, it is incredibly difficult to think positively or feel gratitude for anything because the pain or nausea or weakness can be all-consuming. That said, I also realize that we can always find something to be grateful for, even in the darkest of days. Even if it is as simple as giving thanks for the fact your heart is beating, start there. The frequency of gratitude is just as powerful when you are giving thanks for a penny as it is for being grateful for a million dollars. And just like anything worthwhile, it takes practice.

. . . .

Transcending with Gratitude

When a person shows up in a doctor's office and they're given the diagnosis of rheumatoid arthritis or MS or cancer or diabetes, once they hear that diagnosis, the common emotions they experience are either fear or sadness. They can think positively all they want. They can say, "I'm going to overcome this condition," but if they are feeling fear, that thought never makes it past the brain stem into the body, because it's not in alignment with the body's emotional state. You get that person to change their emotional state and get them into a state of gratitude. Why gratitude? Well, we normally give thanks when we get something.

If you're giving thanks in a state of gratitude, your body believes it is receiving something, because the emotional signature of gratitude means it's already happened. So, the more that we can feel the feeling as if our healing has already occurred, giving thanks for that healing already being present, that is the trigger for our bodies to grow the nerve cells to make the connections to trigger the brain chemistry to reflect that healing.

—Dr. Joe Dispenza

Gratitude Tip

Become aware of where your thoughts start spiraling off to and bring them back to gratitude. This in itself can be a form of meditation. Keep a running list of the things you are grateful for, and start giving thanks for things you want as if you already have them. It might sound something like this: *I am so grateful for my perfect health and the energy to play with my children again.* Or, *I am so grateful now that I am healed, am medication-free, and my pain is completely gone.* Accompany these thoughts with visuals of what that looks like, feeling gratitude and joy as if these were already true. After all, those potentials do exist in the field of infinite possibilities, and according to the experts in this book and great sages of ancient wisdom, gratitude and belief can help you call those experiences in.

"Therefore I tell you, whatever you ask for in prayer, believe that you have received it, and it will be yours."

—Mark 11:24

Growing up Catholic, I was raised to believe in the teachings of the Bible, notably this verse in Matthew 18:20: "For where two or three are gathered in my name, there I am with them." I always believed this to mean that when two or more people are gathered and praying for the same thing, that the power of the prayer is greater. An example of this was Elizabeth's experience in the emergency room in chapter 5, waking up to realize that a hundred people were simultaneously praying for her on Facebook.

In 2008, I took a class at Agape International Spiritual Center taught by Michael B. Beckwith, who shared a story that has stuck with me to this day. He spoke about his enthusiasm for remission and healing in cases where there was absolutely no hope—and then, for whatever reason, there was regeneration. One of the examples he gave was about a woman who had asked her class to pray for her to be placed higher on a kidney transplant list. Beckwith asked her, "Why don't we just pray to heal the kidney you have?" and she said, "No, no, the doctors say this is a very rare disease and can't be cured."

The woman argued with Beckwith about what to pray for until he suggested the following exercise. He asked the class, "How many of you woke up today and gave thanks that your kidneys were working?" Nobody raised their hand. And then he told them that each time they used the restroom throughout the day, they were to give thanks for their kidneys, and to pray for the woman for her perfect kidneys. To her, he said, "I want you to look at all the other organs in your body that are working, and give thanks for them." He also asked her to read a section on kidneys in the health textbook *The Science of*

Mind by Ernest Holmes each day. And he remarked, "While you're giving thanks for the rest of your body parts, you can stay open to the possibility of healing. It may or may not work. I don't have any attachment to this."

A month or so later, the woman announced in class that her kidneys had spontaneously started working again. She didn't need a kidney transplant after all. Beckwith reported that the experience inspired her to adopt a healthier lifestyle, and more than a decade later, her kidneys were still working. This story ties in both the gratitude work that Joe Dispenza and Gregg Braden spoke of, and the concept of "where two or more are gathered." Group intention and prayer make the vision stronger and more powerful!

- -

The Power of Prayer

How could my prayer, how could my meditation, how could my loving thoughts of gratitude and appreciation possibly impact the healing of another person in the room with me or halfway around the world? The answer is that we are deeply connected through a phenomenon that is known as *entanglement*. Entanglement is the term in physics that tells us once something is unified, once something begins as a whole, even though it is separated physically by many miles or light years, energetically everything's still connected. Why is that important? Because if we go back far enough in time, there was a point in time when you, me, and the Earth were all connected, before what is called the big bang, the big release of energy. When that happened physically, particles began to separate; energetically the particles remained connected. We are part of this earth and we are part of one another. And that empowers you and it empowers me to participate in the healing of our bodies and those of our loved ones in ways that science is only beginning to understand.

—**Gregg Braden**

Faith is an aspect of consciousness. People say, "Well, I don't have faith." Actually, everyone has faith of some kind. You either have faith in possibility or you have faith that that possibility doesn't exist. **In a way, we have more faith in the power of cancer to kill us than we have faith in the power of God, the power of miracles, the power of infinite possibility, the power of any force other than what our eyes can see and our hands can touch to actually interrupt the power and the trajectory of disease.**

—**Marianne Williamson**

Joe Dispenza incorporates group intention into his advanced healing workshops. The participants practice meditating and "getting beyond themselves," creating heart-brain coherence with elevated emotions for the first part of the week. At the end of the week they break up into groups of eight, and each group surrounds a person who is most in need of healing. They affectionately call this group setup "the cage." The people that make up the cage of healing are guided into meditation, and once they have quieted their minds and brought their hearts and brains into a beautiful state of coherence, they place their hands that are emitting that coherent energy into the field of the person lying down in the middle of the group.

Joe reports seeing some remarkable results during these group healings. People have gotten up out of wheelchairs, stage IV cancer has healed, blind people have seen again, deaf people have had their hearing restored, and tumors have disappeared. And the time spent sending energy to the person is only about ten minutes. Joe explained to me, "Witnessing a dramatic healing once is a miracle, twice is a coincidence, but what we are seeing over and over are people getting reset back to health with no exogenous substance. It's just energy. And when it happens over and over, there must be a scientific explanation." He went on to tell me about the work of late Yale researcher Harold Saxton Burr and his discoveries about the electromagnetic field of living organisms. Burr's research concluded that it is not matter that emits a field; it is the energetic signature of the field that organizes and creates matter. Thus when you change the field, you change the matter.

What's even more fascinating is that the senders of the intention and energy also experience deep healings, because they are transforming their energy into high-vibration coherent states. What an awesome demonstration of the famous line from the prayer of St. Francis, "For it is in giving that we receive."

Entanglement, quantum physics, and holy books such as the Bible each have their own interpretation of why prayer and intention work. People visit holy sites around the world to receive healing from energy vortexes, healers, mystics, and holy waters. The healing waters of Lourdes, holy sites in India, or other religious sites that people trek to—I don't think we can ever really know if it is the power of belief (the placebo effect) that is responsible for the healing, or if there is an actual miracle from God occurring. All I know is that wherever your faith is strongest, it will lead to your greatest healing.

Whether it is faith in medicine, faith in God, or faith in the incredible healing capacity of the body, you should seek out the treatment where your belief in possibility is the strongest. For some that might mean opting for chemo and radiation (although I recommend taking a look at the nine key factors on page 36 to heal the mental, emotional, and spiritual aspects before, during, or after your conventional treatment). For others it might mean quitting your stressful job, traveling to a holy healing site, or investing in an advanced healing workshop mentioned in this book.

Follow your heart, listen to your intuition, and you will never go astray. As Marianne Williamson reminds us, "Ask in your heart, and the books will fall at your feet."

"What you seek is seeking you."

—Rumi

Chapter 7 Takeaways

- Ancient practices such as yoga and meditation are relatively cost-free ways to help bring our bodies back into balance. Science is proving that these aren't just spiritual practices but that they have real, quantifiable, beneficial physiological effects on the body as well.
- There are many forms of meditation. When practiced regularly, meditation is one of the most powerful tools for physical and spiritual transformation.

- Visualization and using our imagination can activate our innate healing mechanism to help us recover and rehabilitate from all kinds of injuries and conditions, as well as help with pain reduction.
- By combining intention with an elevated emotion, we can cause an effect in order to manifest a desired result. This new model says you have to feel wholeness in order for your healing to occur.
- Gratitude is a powerful creative force and a great tool to help you move out of fear. The more we can give thanks for our healing as if it has already occurred, the more our bodies will make the connections to reflect that healing.
- Wherever your faith is strongest, that will lead to your greatest healing.
- We are all connected and part of one another, and that empowers us to participate in the healing of one another's bodies. Group intention and prayer make the impact stronger and more powerful.

Conclusion

Our bodies are in a constant state of growth and regeneration. We can see this happening clearly in babies as they grow and mature from infancy to adulthood. We can also see it when our hair and nails grow and our skin heals from scrapes or bruises. In fact, our entire body is constantly experiencing regrowth and rebirth from within, with different systems regenerating at different speeds. Your skeleton cells are dying and growing anew, but it takes about ten years for your entire skeleton to be replaced. Your stomach and intestinal lining replace themselves every five days due to the daily wear and tear of digestion. You get an entire new set of skin cells every two to four weeks. Your entire liver is replaced with new liver cells every three hundred to five hundred days, and all of your red blood cells are replaced approximately every one hundred twenty days.

If all of these old cells die and are being replaced by brand-new healthy cells, then why are we chronically sick and diseased?

The answer may lie in our consciousness. Our new healthy cells are responding to the mind-set, emotions, and beliefs we have about our body and our life. Remember what Bruce Lipton taught us about our perception of life and the inner environment we create for our cells. If we are telling our new cells "I am sick" or "I have cancer," simply put, the new cells will adopt that chemistry and perpetuate that story. We need to rip off those labels and stop affirming what we don't want. It's easier said than done, because when we are in fear our minds tend to fixate on the worst-case scenario, and it is hard to break free from the identification with our present circumstance. But by understanding that everything is energy, including the words we speak and the thoughts we think, we can start to imagine a different possibility and tell a new story.

Telling Your Cells a New Story

What you think about and what you talk about is what you create for yourself. Your body creates new cells every day. Stop telling your body what you don't want and start telling your body what you do want, and see what happens. Don't let somebody else put a label on you that says "I have cancer" or "I have MS," and then walk around reaffirming that as fact every day. If that's not what you want, take the label off. It's your body. When you wake up in the morning, say hello to all those new cells. "Thank you for my perfect, healthy life. My body is strong and healthy. I am grateful. I'm abundant."

—**Rob Wergin**

Remember that our body is in activity. In fact, there's only activity in the universe; nothing stands still, except maybe in a museum. The Greek philosopher Heraclitus said, "No man can step into the same river twice," because it's a new man and it's a new river. You cannot step into the same body twice—because every moment you're eating, breathing, digesting, metabolizing, inhaling, exhaling, thinking, and experiencing the world—your body is in activity. If you want to change your body then you have to transcend to that level which is beyond memory, and then you can introduce new, joyful memories that can outshine the traumatic ones. Then you have a chance of reinventing your body. You reinvent your body by resurrecting your soul. There's no other way.

—Deepak Chopra, MD

. . . .

If our beliefs about the state of our body and the negative labels we affirm over and over in our mind inform the new cells that are being born in our bodies every day, we could theoretically perpetuate the disease into a chronic condition. But if we start integrating new belief systems, like Anita Moorjani did (see chapter 2), those new beliefs naturally inform the new cells in a new way, and our bodies will start living a new story.

One way to pivot off the negative story, the pain, and the current limitations is to tap into our feelings of love and gratitude and create more joyful memories, which will begin to overshadow the traumas of the past. A good way to do this is to realign with our purpose, and listen to the calling in our heart—and follow that. Do the things that you may have put aside in order to work, tend to the responsibilities of life, and live up to the expectations of others. Far too often, people wait until they're faced with a life-or-death situation to quit their stressful job, spend more time with their family, appreciate the little miracles in life, do the things that make their heart sing, and start to take advantage of their "last days." And that is precisely when they often spontaneously start to heal.

Let's not wait for a devastating diagnosis to tap into our inner consciousness and live the life we are meant to live! We can make choices every day, no matter how big or small, that allow us to connect our minds, hearts, and spirits with our physical bodies and support a more meaningful, fulfilling life. Whether you are facing a daunting diagnosis now, dealing with unfavorable symptoms, or you simply want to do your best to prevent serious health conditions in the future, start becoming aware of the beliefs you hold and the stories you tell yourself. Take time for self-care, and be aware of what your body is communicating to you. Start quieting your mind and listening to that voice within, your intuition. And remember, your cells are listening to the thoughts in your head and the words you speak out loud, so start telling them a different story. It may feel silly at first, but like any transformational process, it takes practice and commitment. It's easy for our minds to fall back into the loop of negative, fearful thinking, so we need to grab the reins every day and start teaching our minds to go in the positive direction we desire. Only then can our cells and biology follow suit.

How fast can this shift take place? While healing occurs differently for everyone, David Hamilton told me a fascinating story that demonstrates just how quickly and powerfully our consciousness can affect our physiology. He explained to me that there is a psychological condition called dissociative identity disorder (DID), which used to be called multiple personality disorder. When a person with DID moves into a completely different personality, what follows are sometimes actual and instantaneous changes in their biology. In one well-known case, a woman with DID said that one of her distinct personalities was allergic to orange juice. In the presence of a psychiatrist she drank orange juice, and hives, an allergic reaction, appeared on her arm. Moments later, in front of the same psychiatrist, as her personality shifted to a different one who was not allergic to citrus, the hives disappeared in a matter of seconds.

Joe Dispenza teaches us that our personality, which stems from our beliefs about life, shapes our personal reality. As David Hamilton explains, our beliefs can be so powerful that they can facilitate really incredible things—sometimes in an instant!

What are some labels you are carrying that are inform-ing your cells? What is a new story you can tell them? What are three affirmations you can start to tell your-self every morning? For example: I am overflowing with

joy. I feel so energized and alive. I am grateful for my perfect health.

In this book I have outlined how trauma, negative emotions, and subconscious beliefs can all lead to disease, which requires a more holistic approach to healing. But you may wonder about children who come into this world already sick or become ill at a very young age. Surely their conditions can't be a result of accumulated stress or unprocessed trauma or disempowering beliefs. Why do innocent children get sick? Why anyone contracts a disease is beyond the scope of our knowledge. Is it karmic? Is it fate? Did they choose that path before coming into this world as a part of their soul's evolution? Or is it caused by stress, toxicity, or negative subconscious beliefs of the parents while the child is in utero?

. . . .

Why Do Innocent Children Get Sick?

From a spiritual perspective, I see many individuals choosing to come into this world knowing they're going to go through some stuff. They're coming to help others increase their awareness and achieve higher evolution of their soul, individually and collectively as a society. So we shouldn't look at it like,

"Well, this person was born with this disease; what's wrong?" Many of these individuals are coming with very special gifts. On another level, today, a baby that's being born is affected with more toxins than ever.

—Dr. Michael B. Beckwith

We absolutely know—this is not some mystery—we know where a lot of cancers come from: they have to do with chemicals in the food; they have to do with chemicals in the air; they have to do with chemicals in the earth. So did human consciousness create this? Absolutely, but it's not necessarily the consciousness of the person who contracted the disease.

—Marianne Williamson

This is where we begin to cross the boundaries of science and spirituality and words like *karma* or *destiny* or *fate*. What I do know without any shadow of a doubt is once that beautiful child arrives in this world, their bodies, their cells, their DNA will respond to the environment and the conditions that we give to them. Our job is to learn to optimize those environments and those conditions.

—Gregg Braden

. . . .

Whatever the case may be, love, conviction, and awareness are key in helping a child heal. By seven years old, children have downloaded the subconscious beliefs and behaviors of their caretakers. Mothers and fathers must be aware of the emotions they are feeling while the child is developing in utero. We must become conscious of the fears we are expressing and the words we are saying around a child who is diagnosed with a serious condition. We must educate ourselves and apply all the same tools and principles as if it were our own diagnosis. And we must do everything we can to strengthen not only their immune systems but also their belief in possibility. Children are so much closer to the world of spirit than we are, and their imagination is extremely powerful—we must help them tap into that source of strength.

What if someone close to you, child or otherwise, receives a difficult diagnosis or is suffering from a chronic condition? I asked the experts how we as loved ones could further help those in need of guidance and support.

. . . .

Healing Effects of Social Support

Increasing social support was one of the nine key factors for radical remission that I expected to come up. I expected people to say that they felt this outpouring of love from friends and family. What I wasn't expecting was for them to say emphatically that it helped their bodies heal. It's nice to feel loved by your friends and family, but from a scientific standpoint, I wasn't really clear that it could help your body heal. But they were clear: This helped my body fight cancer. And again, I went back to the research that other people have done in randomized control trials, and it is overwhelmingly true that people who have self-perceived strong social support networks live longer, and they just need to believe that they're loved.

If you perceive that people are coming to help you and hold you and help you through this process, and you feel this outpouring of love, they are actually helping your body heal. Because as soon as you believe that people are sending you love, you have an oxytocin response, and oxytocin release has been associated with increased white blood cells, and your immune response just goes through the roof. By bringing food or running errands or sending an email that says "I'm thinking about you," you are literally helping your loved ones heal. **Much of my research has shown me that we have much more power over our life and our health than we previously thought. We are not helpless.** Even doing a little thing will actually help your loved one build a stronger immune system, and that's what they need to heal.

—Kelly Turner, PhD

We now know that people who attend support groups or spiritual support groups live, on average, twice as long after the diagnosis of a life-challenging illness. We know that people who are prayed for get out of intensive care units faster. I think the most important thing that we all need to be in touch with is our own capacity for empathy and compassion. The first thing that you say is that you're sorry. That person who was just diagnosed does not need a lecture. It's interesting because that holy mind, that natural intelligence doesn't ask, "What do I do, what do I say?" It first seeks to be the presence of love and compassion in that person's life. If there's something for you to say, you'll be led from within to say it. There might be a book you recommend, there might be a meditation class you invite that person to. There might be a story that you end up telling them.

Sometimes if a person has just been diagnosed with an illness, it helps that you're going to just sit there with them while they cry, or maybe you even cry with them. Join people in that state of being, which is your own oneness with that person. Words are but symbols. It might be holding someone's hand. It might be, "I'll go to chemo with you."

—Marianne Williamson

• •

Being raised Catholic by parents who came from a long history of faithful churchgoers, I had a childhood fascination with stories from the Bible, of Jesus healing lepers and creating all sorts of miracles. I now know the concept of spontaneous healing applies across any and all religious beliefs. Healing is a universal experience, not claimed by any one religion or medical science, and there is an undeniable connection between the metaphysical, the scientific, and the spiritual.

• •

Seeing beyond the Illusion

Miracles arise from conviction. When Jesus looked at the leper, he saw through the veil of illusion, which is to say he transcended the mere perception of the physical body. He had developed what you could call the vision of the Holy Spirit when he looked at a person and looked past the body, and this is what forgiveness actually is. The whole metaphysical notion here is that spirit is real and matter is not.

Buddha said it's all an illusion, *A Course in Miracles* said it's all an illusion, and Einstein said it: that this whole, physical, three-dimensional reality is just posing as ultimate reality. So your physical body can have leprosy, but your spirit cannot have leprosy. Your spirit is perfect; your spirit is eternal. It cannot get sick and it cannot die. Jesus did not limit his perception to the level of leprosy. He looked beyond it, so he didn't really believe in leprosy. His conviction was so strong that in his presence the leper couldn't believe in leprosy either. As soon as the leper could no longer believe in it, he had a moment where he saw through that illusion himself, and he was healed. Jesus is one whose mind has been healed of the illusion, like Buddha and others.

So the miracle worker is someone who is the presence of the alternative. Our job in any situation is to accept that correction of our perception. Most of us aren't on the level of Jesus or whomever, but *A Course in Miracles* says you can go to the highest level of thinking of which the ego is capable, and God himself will lift you the rest of the way.

—**Marianne Williamson**

How do we bring metaphysical lessons into something more practical and tangible? While we might not be able to demonstrate the inspiring gifts of Jesus, Buddha, and other masters, the truth is that we do all possess our own gifts and the ability to make important contributions in our lifetime. Our unique purpose on this planet is so important that it even affects our health. When we deny our purpose and passion, we resist that natural intelligence within, and as we have learned by now, resistance blocks the flow of energy, causing stagnation and dis-ease.

Realigning with our Passion and Purpose

A radical remission survivor changes their life completely, and the way that they're willing to do that is if they figure out why they want to still live here in this body on this earth. Reconnecting to their reasons for living is huge. For most people it's a desire to be around family, to have kids, or to see their kids grow up. But I also interviewed plenty of people without kids who said, "You know what? I'm actually not afraid of death. I'll go to that other side when it's my time, but in the meantime, I really want to finish that novel. If there's one thing I can leave on this physical planet Earth, it would be that novel." Or it would be "this painting," or "I really want to climb Mount Kilimanjaro before I depart." They connect to these reasons, and that gives them life force, or chi.

One of the traditional Chinese medicine practitioners that I interviewed in Shanghai, China, said that cancer is the depletion of chi. Your chi is leaving your system, and there's not enough coming back in to make you complete or to have your system working well. He said when he works with cancer patients and he's feeling their pulse and looking at their tongue, he notices that they're very deficient in life force. Their chi has been expelled, and it's not coming back in. By reconnecting to your life's purpose, you actually call chi in [to your body], and it fills you up to give you the energy to operate all these systems, including your detoxification system.

—Kelly Turner, PhD

We're all fated to walk a path on this road, and the road is destined to always come to a fork. When I'm standing at the fork I've got two choices. When I choose the safe path, that's when my symptoms begin, because it's a wounding of my spirit. For every percentage point that my spirit is not walking the path that's the best use of me, I am out of step with the universal dance of why I am here. But when I choose the path that's my dharma, that makes the best use of me, it gets my juices flowing and makes me the happiest person in the world, even if it seems like it can't possibly work.

—**Dr. Jeffrey Thompson**

Focus on life. Focus on something that brings you joy. Focus on love, focus on your loved ones, and spend every day doing things that make you feel good. Think of the word *remission* as actually meaning, "Remember my mission." Now it's time for you to go and remember your mission.

—**Anita Moorjani**

. . . .

"There are no incurable diseases,
only incurable people."

—**Bernie Siegel, MD**

I love this quote from Dr. Bernie Siegel. This is not to say that if someone was not able to heal, that they did something wrong. This is not about blame. Healing takes place on many levels and on many timelines, and even if someone may not heal entirely in a physical sense, often they say that they found an unmatched joy, grace, and freedom because they did reconnect with their purpose, their loved ones, or their joy. **Ultimately what I have found is that healing is spiritual.** It's a journey beyond our selves, our egos, our illusions of inadequacy and separation, and back to the wholeness and love of our spirit—who we truly are. According to many spiritual traditions, the key ultimately lies in transcending our fear of death. How better to overcome fear than to embrace love? To return to love, trusting that the universe, that life, that God (whatever term you define Source as) is always for us and never against us. Any challenges we experience along the way are there for the evolution of our souls. And as Anita Moorjani shared with us, the unconditional, indescribable love we may return to after we leave our physical bodies is not something to fear.

Our thoughts, beliefs, and emotions have more impact on our physical health than we realize, and we have more control over our own health and life than we have been taught to believe. I hope this book has inspired you with a new understanding of the miraculous nature of the human body, and the extraordinary capacity for healing within us all. I hope you feel transformative changes from within that connect your mind, body, and spirit. I hope you are empowered to step forward on your own spiritual journey toward better health and a more fulfilling life.

You deserve nothing less than the miracles that are waiting for you in the field of infinite possibilities.

Final Takeaways from Our Experts

Healing is actually a powerful revelation of the essential wholeness that's already within us. We're not adding anything to us; we're basically letting go of that which is covering up the healing. What happens is it feels like a homecoming. You're actually coming home to the essential wholeness you may have had before your mind got cluttered with fear and worry. Healing is really wholeness being revealed.

—**Dr. Michael B. Beckwith**

I think we can't just say, "Dear God, heal my cancer" or "Dear God, heal my diabetes." We must say, "Dear God, heal my life; dear God, heal my heart." I know many people who have contracted very serious, even life-threatening illnesses who have come to feel, even in instances where their bodies did not heal, that other parts of them did heal. And in some cases they found love, joy, and happiness beyond what they had known before.

—**Marianne Williamson**

When I think of everything that we know today and the wisdom of five thousand years of our ancestors before today, what it tells me at the deepest level of our existence is simply this: the better we know ourselves, the better equipped we are to embrace whatever it is that life brings to our doorstep.

—Gregg Braden

There's not a human being on the planet who doesn't see a newborn baby and intuitively feel the preciousness of that . . . But at some point you decided that you weren't that precious anymore. That's when abuse started. If I could get people to realize how precious they are and realize they're an expression of life . . . There is no other you out there. That's one in eight billion, that's pretty special. I guarantee you most people don't give themselves that kind of love and care. That would be a wonderful precursor to healing.

—Peter Crone

My one takeaway message for healing would be to educate yourself about the mind-body connection, because your mind exerts an extraordinarily powerful effect on your body twenty-four hours a day, 365 days a year. If we educate ourselves on how that occurs, how that works, then we can actually start to harness the mind/body connection by choosing what direction to focus our minds in.

—David R. Hamilton, PhD

The reason I do this research is because every day I meet someone who beat incredible odds and turned around stage IV cancer. And if they can do it, and if I meet new people every day who are doing it, then at some point we all can do it. And that's hopeful. We may not know exactly how to do it yet. We may not know exactly what you should do to achieve what they did. But the simple fact that they exist, and are existing more and more, makes me realize that healing can really happen at any time. Even when you're at "death's door," you can still turn things around. And that's inspiring to me.

—Kelly Turner, PhD

You're a participant in your own healing, so get to know more about what you have than your doctor [knows]. Go Google search or look up the National Library of Medicine. Do a PubMed search and take in everything that's there—some of it useful, some of it not, but you will intuitively know what makes sense for you. Then explore everything in mind/body medicine, spiritual healing, and the world of herbs and diet and food and medicine and environment: all the things that create experience of life. And ultimately go beyond your fear of death, because death happens to an experience, not to you.

—**Deepak Chopra, MD**

Your body loves you. It loves you unconditionally, and it's not letting you down. Have patience, have compassion. Take one day at a time. You're going to get there. It doesn't matter how long you've been sick; you can heal. Always remember that.

—**Anthony William**

It's my passionate belief that every single person has within them the potential to transform their experience, not just alleviate symptoms. Not just get rid of the headache or have a bit more energy or sleep a bit better. But really transform your experience into one of self-agency, into one of purpose, and to one of a sense of connectedness to this web that already exists. It's just a matter of really waking up to it and feeling held by it. That's the beauty and promise of true healing. It's something that, unfortunately, the conventional model doesn't even really put on the menu. It's my expectation that this will become more and more compelling to more and more people as we all grow together into a different kind of medicine.

—Kelly Brogan, MD

I think one of the most important aspects of understanding our life and our health is that we are not victims of our genetics, as we have been programmed to believe. Because as victims it says you are powerless, which leads to irresponsibility. "Well if I can't control it, then why do I even care about doing anything about it?" What we need to understand is we are in absolute control. We can change anything in our biology. You could be terminally sick with cancer, like my dear friend Anita Moorjani. Anita had an out-of-body experience and she realized that her cultural programming conflicted with her life, and that conflict led to the illness. By resolving these conflicts, she came back from a place that her oncologist says nobody comes back from. Change the belief and you can come back from death.

—Bruce Lipton, PhD

Life is not a perfect; life is a practice. What would it be like to have a practice of being healthy? Healthy people have healthy habits. Rather than this being something that you just read in a book, put it into action. Fall down. Get back up. Lean into it, dig deeper, go for it. Be courageous. Reach out to other people and ask them their stories. Don't ever give up.

—**Dr. Darren Weissman**

The big takeaway about healing? Anything is possible. Hope is your biggest ally. When you love yourself, when you truly love yourself, you recognize that you're quite a magical being. When you heal your past and get rid of all the stuff that's bothering you, you find that healing happens, and it feels so wonderful. It feels like you're light as a feather.

—**Joan Borysenko, PhD**

I think when we take time out of our busy lives to invest in ourselves—to become a work in progress, to begin to decide what thoughts we no longer want to think, what behaviors we'd like to change, what emotions we want to transform, and every single day make an effort to remove the blocks and the masks, the facades that stop the flow of the divine in us—when we begin to do that kind of work, that divine intelligence begins to move through us. And this is the time in history—right now—where people are looking for answers. And they secretly believe in themselves. And I think that belief in ourselves and belief in infinite possibilities makes life really exciting. So when our will matches the will of the divine intelligence within us, when our mind matches its mind, and when our love for life matches its love for life, I think it always answers the call.

—**Dr. Joe Dispenza**

Acknowledgments

First and foremost I would like to thank my loving husband for supporting me throughout the process of making the *Heal* documentary and writing this book. His unwavering belief in me gave me the courage to follow my heart and realize this passion and vision of mine. His encouragement and trust gave me the guts to take risks and follow my dream. Words cannot express my gratitude for you, AG.

Because this book is a direct result of the film, I'd like to start by thanking all of the wonderful, dedicated people who made the film possible. Deep gratitude for my producing partner Adam Schomer, who believed in my vision the whole way through and always supported my instincts, despite it being my first time directing. His genuine passion for helping people, his tireless work ethic, his sense of humor in challenging times, and his experience in conscious filmmaking helped make it all possible. Thank you to Richell Morrissey for all of her support and contribution as a creative producer in the early stages. Thank you to Christopher Gallo and Ana Amortegui, whose cinematography made the film so incredibly beautiful. Gallo, thank you for teaching me to trust my intuition and helping me find my power, while also showing me the world through a stunning new lens. Ana, thank you for being pure joy and light to work with. A big thank-you to Tina Mascara, the brilliant editor, for her powerful storytelling and great attitude at the end of a long day. Deep gratitude to Michael Mollura for creating the most beautiful original music for *Heal* under an impossibly tight timeline and budget. A big thanks also to Mark DeNicola and Ginger Pullman, my genius social media team, for their commitment to and passion for the *Heal* movement. And a very sincere thanks to the rest of the crewmembers along the way, who put their heart and soul into the diligent work they contributed. Salima Ruffin, thank you for being a wonderful cheerleader and powerful connector. To Connie Ruvalcaba and Andy McBride, thank you both for all of your moral support and seamless accounting throughout the making of *Heal*. Jessica Duncan, thank you for assisting me and the *Heal* team with everything from life-saving coffee runs to all the other major things you helped us with. And to Matthew DeNicola and Scott Burroughs, thank you for your diligent legal work every step of the way. Finally, to Jim Martin and our team at the Orchard, who believed in *Heal* from the beginning and agreed that the message needed to be heard around the globe, thank you so much.

Neither the film nor the book would've been possible without the gracious participation of all of the esteemed *Heal* experts. I am eternally grateful not only for all they have taught me personally over the years but also for the kindness and generosity they exuded during the sometimes tedious filming process. Michael B. Beckwith, Gregg Braden, Kelly Brogan, Joan Borysenko, Deepak Chopra, Peter Crone, Joe Dispenza, David Hamilton, Bruce Lipton, Anita Moorjani, Patti Penn, Dianne Porchia, Bernie Siegel, Jeffrey Thompson, Kelly Turner, Darren Weissman, Rob Wergin, Anthony William, and Marianne Williamson, thank you so much for your dedication to sharing your message and for making the world a more enlightened, loving place. Your continued support of *Heal* warms my soul, and I feel incredibly blessed to have been able to work with and learn from each and every one of you. Also, a big thank-you to all of the amazing executive assistants, directors, and teams of experts who made this process such an effortless and joyful experience.

To Eva Lee and Elizabeth Craig, I cannot express enough how deeply I admire your bravery and generosity in sharing your incredibly personal healing journeys with me and the *Heal* audience. I wish you both all the prosperity and perfect health that life has to offer. Thank you for being my favorite parts of *Heal*.

I am deeply grateful for my publishing team at Beyond Words, who have all been so patient, supportive, and nurturing throughout the writing process. Richard and Michele Cohn, you are incredible partners, and it's so refreshing to work with such good, honest, brilliant people. The rest of the team at Beyond Words, including Emily Einolander, Lindsay Easterbrooks-Brown, Linda Meyer, Emmalisa Sparrow Wood, Devon Smith, Corinne Kalasky, Tara Lehmann, and Cindy Nickles, I thank you for your hard work. And finally a big thank you to freelancers Emily Han for her insight, experience, and thoughtful, lyrical editing, and Linda Sivertsen for her genius input and support.

I'd like to especially thank Ursula Cary, who gently and enthusiastically held my hand throughout the entire writing process (while we both navigated different stages of pregnancy, no less!). She helped me finish the book just in time for her to go into labor with her second child. You are truly a superwoman, UC! Thank you, Lori Bregman, for introducing us! And I'd like to say another big thank-you to Joe Dispenza, who somehow found the time during his incredibly busy speaking schedule and workshop calendar to write such a thoughtful and powerful foreword.

Last but not least, I'd like to thank my tribe of friends and family who are always there to cheer me on, celebrate life's little triumphs with, and walk beside me during difficult times. To my beautiful mom, Sandy; hilarious dad, Marty; and genius brother, Ryan—all of whom I love more than the world—thank you for being my endless power source of unconditional love and support. Words cannot express how blessed I am to have you as my foundation and biggest cheerleaders. To Carolyn, my best friend, who always lifts me up, while still managing to keep me grounded in truth and humility—Oatpan emails for life! To my close girlfriends, a bunch of badass women who inspire me every day with their hearts, minds, accomplishments, and unwavering support of one another (you know who you are), thank you for your true friendship. To Amy, my sis-in-law, and my angel of a nephew, Declan, thank you for the light you bring to my life. And to my mother-in-law, Tata Marie Gores, thank you for raising such an amazing son and continuing to be such an incredibly strong and loving role model for us all.

And to all of you on a healing path who have turned to this book for inspiration and knowledge, thank you for trusting me to curate the empowering wisdom from the experts and the inspiring real-life stories I've included in *Heal*. May God bless you on your journey.

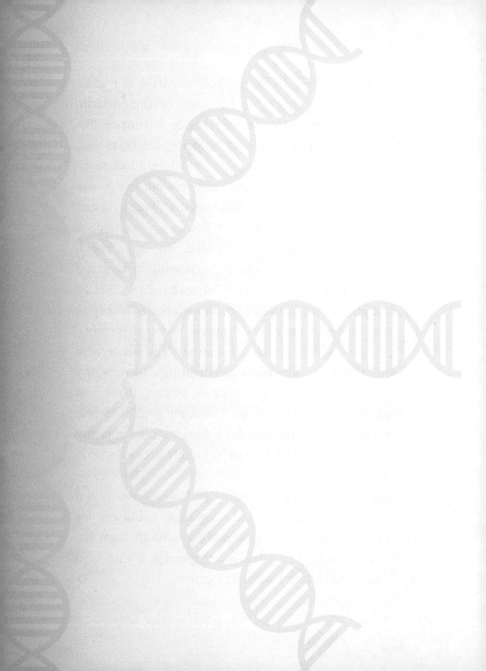

Daily Reminders for Your Healing Journey

Now that you have flipped the switch "on" and discovered the powerful healer within you, here are ten daily reminders to help support you on your journey. You can choose one to focus on and implement each day or read through all ten—each reminder is designed to help deepen your awareness and activate your greatest potential. You may want to photocopy these pages and keep posted somewhere handy, or copy the reminders into your journal to spark inspiration and greater exploration.

1. Become aware of your thoughts, beliefs, and emotions, as they have an extremely powerful effect on your physical health.

2. Accept where you are in the present moment. Only when you accept can you move forward and make new, empowered choices.

3. Believe your diagnosis, but make your own prognosis. Choose the outcome you want out of the field of infinite possibilities, focus on that potential, and trust that the way will appear.

4. Seek a second or third opinion, and surround yourself with positive, supportive friends and practitioners who fuel your hope and belief in possibility.

5. Find ways to tap into the chemistry of love, the greatest healing power of all.

6. Eat a healthy, unprocessed diet as often as possible, and find time to enjoy nature's powerful healing properties.

7. Learn to meditate, even if it means sitting quietly and focusing on your breath for just five minutes a day. Meditation, which can come in many forms, simply requires quieting the mind and allowing the space for intuition and inspiration to arise.

8. Gratitude and forgiveness are two powerful tools for letting go and transcending pain and fear. Practice expressing gratitude for even the smallest things in life that bring you joy. And practice forgiveness to free up the energy needed for healing.

9. Combine visualization and elevated emotion to cause the effect you desire in life. In other words, spend a few minutes every day imagining yourself already healed, while feeling the joy and gratitude of already being healed and doing the things you love again. The feeling creates the healing.

10. Be gentle with yourself and take it one day at a time. Remember, there is always hope.

Notes

1. Wullianallur Raghupathi and Viju Raghugpathi, "An Empirical Study of Chronic Diseases in the United States: A Visual Analytics Approach to Public Heath," *International Journal of Environmental Research and Public Health* 15, no. 3 (March 2018): 431, https://www.ncbi.nlm.nih .gov/pmc/articles/PMC5876976/.

2. Susanna Schrobsdorff, "Teen Depression and Anxiety: Why the Kids Are Not Alright," *Time*, October 26, 2016, http://time.com/4547322 /american-teens-anxious-depressed-overwhelmed/.

3. Ramin Mojtabai, Mark Olfson, and Beth Han, "National Trends in the Prevalence and Treatment of Depression in Adolescents and Young Adults," *Pediatrics* 138, no. 6 (December 2016), http://pediatrics.aappub lications.org/content/pediatrics/138/6/e20161878.full.pdf.

4. Jean M. Twenge, "Time Period and Birth Cohort Differences in Depressive Symptoms in the U.S., 1982–2013," *Social Indicators Research* 121,

no. 2 (April 2015): 437, https://link.springer.com/article/10.1007/s11205-014-0647-1.

5. "About Genetically Engineered Foods," Center for Food Safety (website), accessed December 15, 2018, https://www.centerforfoodsafety.org/issues/311/ge-foods/about-ge-foods.

6. "About Chronic Diseases," National Health Council, last modified July 29, 2014, http://www.nationalhealthcouncil.org/sites/default/files/NHC_Files/Pdf_Files/AboutChronicDisease.pdf.

7. "Heath and Economic Costs of Chronic Diseases," National Center for Chronic Disease Prevention and Health Promotion, last modified February 11, 2019, https://www.cdc.gov/chronicdisease/about/costs/index.htm.

8. Masaru Emoto, *The Hidden Messages in Water*, trans. David A Thayne (Hillsboro, OR: Beyond Words Publishing, 2004), 39.

9. Emoto, *Hidden Messages in Water*, 43.

10. Ariana Eunjung Cha, "Researchers: Medical Errors Now Third Leading Cause of Death in United States," *Washington Post*, May 3, 2016, https://www.washingtonpost.com/news/to-your-health/wp/2016/05/03/researchers-medical-errors-now-third-leading-cause-of-death-in-united-states/.

11. "Medical Hypnosis," Stanford Health Care, accessed March 7, 2019, https://stanfordhealthcare.org/medical-treatments/c/complementary-medicine/types/medical-hypnosis.html.

12. "Everything You Need to Know about the Ketogenic Diet," Mercola .com, accessed May 7, 2019, https://www.mercola.com/calendar/2018 /keto.htm.

13. Deborah Franklin, "How Hospital Gardens Help Patients Heal," *Scientific American*, March 1, 2012, https://www.scientificamerican .com/article/nature-that-nurtures/.

14. Insook Lee et al., "Effects of Forest Therapy on Depressive Symptoms among Adults: A Systematic Review," *International Journal of Environmental Research and Public Health* 14, no. 3 (March 2017): 321, https:// www.researchgate.net/publication/315474109_Effects_of_Forest _Therapy_on_Depressive_Symptoms_among_Adults_A_Systematic _Review.

15. Céline Cousteau, foreword to *Blue Mind: The Surprising Science That Shows How Being Near, In, On, or Under Water Can Make You Happier, Healthier, More Connected, and Better at What You Do*, by Wallace J. Nichols (New York: Little, Brown, 2014).

16. Sharon Begley, "The Brain: How the Brain Rewires Itself," *Time*, January 19, 2007, http://content.time.com/time/magazine/article/0,9171 ,1580438,00.html.

17. "Virtual Reality Pain Reduction," Human Photonics Laboratory, University of Washington, accessed January 2, 2019, https://depts .washington.edu/hplab/research/virtual-reality/.

Further Reading

Michael Bernard Beckwith

Life Visioning: A Transformative Process for Activating Your Unique Gifts and Highest Potential (Sounds True, 2011).

Joan Borysenko

Minding the Body, Mending the Mind (Da Capo, 2007).

Gregg Braden

The Divine Matrix: Bridging Time, Space, Miracles, and Belief (Hay House, 2006).

Human by Design: From Evolution by Chance to Transformation by Choice (Penguin Random House, 2017).

The Spontaneous Healing of Belief: Shattering the Paradigm of False Limits (Hay House, 2008).

Kelly Brogan

A Mind of Your Own: The Truth about Depression and How Women Can Heal Their Bodies to Reclaim Their Lives (HarperCollins, 2016).

Rhonda Byrne

The Secret (Beyond Words/Atria Books, 2006).

Kris Carr

Crazy Sexy Cancer Tips (Skirt!, 2007).

Deepak Chopra

Perfect Health: The Complete Mind/Body Guide (Harmony Books, 1991).

Quantum Healing: Exploring the Frontiers of Mind/Body Medicine (Bantam Books, 2015).

Deepak Chopra and Rudolph E. Tanzi

The Healing Self: A Revolutionary New Plan to Supercharge Your Immunity and Stay Well for Life (Harmony Books, 2018).

Joe Dispenza

Becoming Supernatural: How Common People Are Doing the Uncommon (Hay House, 2017).

Breaking the Habit of Being Yourself: How to Lose Your Mind and Create a New One (Hay House, 2013).

You Are the Placebo: Making Your Mind Matter (Hay House, 2014).

Wayne W. Dyer

Change Your Thoughts, Change Your Life: Living the Wisdom of the Tao (Hay House, 2007).

The Power of Intention: Learning to Co-create Your World Your Way (Hay House, 2004).

Wishes Fulfilled: Mastering the Art of Manifesting (Hay House, 2012).

Masaru Emoto

The Healing Power of Water (Hay House, 2008).

The Hidden Messages in Water (Beyond Words Publishing, 2004).

Water Crystal Healing: Music and Images to Restore Your Well-Being (Atria Books, 2006).

Jennifer Giustra-Kozek

Healing without Hurting: Treating ADHD, Apraxia, and Autism Spectrum Disorders Naturally and Effectively without Harmful Medications (Changing Lives Press, 2014).

David R. Hamilton

The Five Side Effects of Kindness: This Book Will Make You Feel Better, Be Happier, and Live Longer (Hay House, 2017).

How Your Mind Can Heal Your Body (Hay House UK, 2008).

I Heart Me: The Science of Self-Love (Hay House UK, 2015).

David R. Hawkins

Letting Go: The Pathway of Surrender (Hay House, 2014).

Power vs. Force: The Hidden Determinants of Human Behavior (Hay House, 2014).

Louise Hay

You Can Heal Your Life (Hay House, 1984).

Ernest Holmes

The Science of the Mind: The Complete Edition (Penguin Group, 1950).

Bruce Lipton

The Biology of Belief: Unleashing the Power of Consciousness, Matter, and Miracles (Hay House, 2005).

The Honeymoon Effect: The Science of Creating Heaven on Earth (Hay House, 2013).

Lynne McTaggart

The Field: The Quest for the Secret Force of the Universe (HarperCollins, 2008).

The Power of Eight: Harnessing the Miraculous Energy of a Small Group to Heal Others, Your Life, and the World (Atria Books, 2017).

Caroline Myss

Anatomy of the Spirit: The Seven Stages of Power and Healing (Harmony Books, 1996).

Wallace J. Nichols

Blue Mind: The Surprising Science That Shows How Being Near, In, On, or Under Water Can Make You Happier, Healthier, More Connected, and Better at What You Do (Little, Brown, 2014).

Florence Scovel Shinn

The Game of Life and How to Play It (DeVorss & Company, 1979).

Bernie S. Siegel

Peace, Love, and Healing: Bodymind Communication and the Path to Self-Healing; An Exploration (HarperPerennial, 1998).

Kelly A. Turner

Radical Remission: Surviving Cancer against All Odds (HarperOne, 2014).

Darren R. Weissman

The Power of Infinite Love and Gratitude: An Evolutionary Journey to Awakening Your Spirit (Hay House, 2007).

Robert Whitaker

Anatomy of an Epidemic: Magic Bullets, Psychiatric Drugs, and the Astonishing Rise of Mental Illness in America (Crown, 2010).

Anthony William

Medical Medium: Secrets behind Chronic and Mystery Illness and How to Finally Heal (Hay House, 2015).

Medical Medium Life-Changing Foods: Save Yourself and the Ones You Love with the Hidden Healing Powers of Fruits and Vegetables (Hay House, 2016).

Medical Medium Liver Rescue: Answers to Eczema, Psoriasis, Diabetes, Strep, Acne, Gout, Bloating, Gallstones, Adrenal Stress, Fatigue, Fatty Liver, Weight Issues, SIBO, and Autoimmune Disease (Hay House, 2018).

Medical Medium Thyroid Healing: The Truth behind Hashimoto's, Graves', Insomnia, Hypothyroidism, Thyroid Nodules, and Epstein-Barr (Hay House, 2017).

Florence Williams

The Nature Fix: Why Nature Makes Us Happier, Healthier, and More Creative (W. W. Norton, 2017).

Marianne Williamson

A Return to Love: Reflections on the Principles of "A Course in Miracles" (HarperPerennial, 1996).

Tears to Triumph: Spiritual Healing for the Modern Plagues of Anxiety and Depression (HarperCollins, 2016).

Meet the
Experts

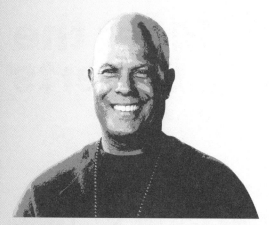

Dr. Michael Bernard Beckwith

Founder of Agape International Spiritual Center, Author

In 1986, Dr. Michael Bernard Beckwith founded the Agape International Spiritual Center, a trans-denominational community of thousands of local members and global live streamers. His organization is highly regarded for its cultural, racial, and spiritual diversity. Dr. Beckwith is a sought-after meditation teacher, conference speaker, and seminar leader on the Life Visioning Process, which he originated. Three of his most recent books, *Life Visioning*, *Spiritual Liberation*, and *TranscenDance Expanded*, are recipients of the prestigious Nautilus Award. He has appeared in his own PBS special, *The Answer Is You*, and on his radio show, *Wake Up: The Sound of Transformation*.

www.michaelbernardbeckwith.com

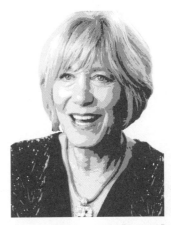

Joan Borysenko, PhD

Psychoneuroimmunologist, President of MindBody Health Services

Dr. Joan Borysenko is a distinguished pioneer in integrative medicine and a world-renowned expert in the mind-body connection. In the early 1980s, Dr. Borysenko cofounded a mind-body clinic, became licensed as a psychologist, and was appointed instructor in medicine at the Harvard Medical School. Her years of clinical experience and research culminated in the 1987 publication of the *New York Times* bestseller *Minding the Body, Mending the Mind*. She is the author or coauthor of thirteen other books and numerous audio and video programs, including the public television special *Inner Peace for Busy People*. She is also the founding partner of Mind/Body Health Sciences, LLC, located in Boulder, Colorado, and the director of the Claritas Institute Interspiritual Mentor Training Program.

www.joanborysenko.com

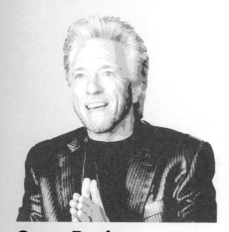

Gregg Braden

Geologist, *New York Times* Bestselling Author

Gregg Braden is internationally renowned as a pioneer in bridging science, spirituality, and the real world. Following a successful career as a computer geologist during the 1970s energy crisis, he worked as a senior liaison with the US Air Force Space Command during the Cold War years of the 1980s. Since 1986 Gregg has explored high-mountain villages, remote monasteries, and forgotten texts to merge their timeless secrets with the best science of today. His discoveries have led to eleven award-winning books published in thirty-eight languages. Gregg has received numerous honors for his work, including a 2016 nomination for the prestigious Templeton Award.

www.greggbraden.com

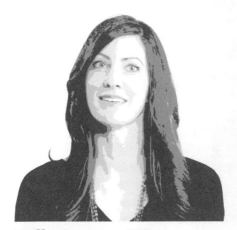

Kelly Brogan, MD
Holistic Psychiatrist,
New York Times Bestselling Author

Dr. Kelly Brogan is a Manhattan-based holistic women's health psychiatrist, author of the *New York Times* bestselling book *A Mind of Your Own*, and coeditor of the landmark textbook *Integrative Therapies for Depression*. She completed her psychiatric training and fellowship at NYU Medical Center after graduating from Cornell University Medical College, and has a BS from MIT in systems neuroscience. Dr. Brogan is board certified in psychiatry, psychosomatic medicine, and integrative holistic medicine, and is specialized in a root-cause resolution approach to psychiatric syndromes and symptoms. She is a certified KRI Kundalini Yoga teacher and a mother of two.

www.kellybroganmd.com

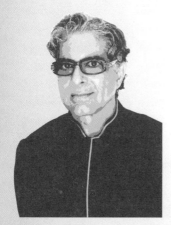

Deepak Chopra, MD, FACP
New York Times Bestselling Author, Speaker

A world-renowned pioneer in integrative medicine and personal transformation, Dr. Deepak Chopra is the founder of the Chopra Foundation and cofounder of Jiyo.com and the Chopra Center for Wellbeing. *Time* magazine has described Dr. Chopra as "one of the top 100 heroes and icons of the century." Deepak Chopra is board certified in internal medicine, endocrinology, and metabolism; a fellow of the American College of Physicians; and clinical professor in medicine and public health at the University of California, San Diego. The *World Post* and *Huffington Post* global internet survey ranked Chopra "#17 influential thinker in the world" and "#1 in Medicine." He is the author of more than eighty-five books, including twenty-five *New York Times* bestsellers.

www.chopra.com

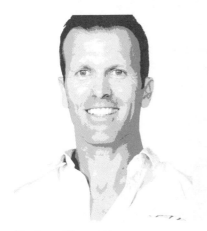

Peter Crone

Mind and Performance Coach, Ayurveda Practitioner

Born and raised in England, where he received both his bachelor's and master's degrees with honors, Peter is an internationally recognized mind/body wellness coach, spiritual teacher, and life transformation expert. On completing his thesis, he moved to the United States and spent more than five years as an exclusive trainer to some of Hollywood's biggest stars. When working with the body he is unrivaled, basing his training on an incredible foundation of knowledge in Ayurveda, human biology, exercise physiology, biomechanics, and anatomy.

www.bealive.com

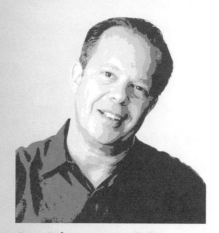

Joe Dispenza, DC

Researcher, *New York Times* Bestselling Author

Dr. Joe Dispenza first caught the public's eye as one of the scientists featured in the award-winning film *What the BLEEP Do We Know!?* Since that movie's release in 2004, Dr. Joe has been invited to speak in more than twenty-seven countries on six continents. In addition to offering a variety of online courses and tele-classes, he personally teaches three-day progressive workshops and five-day advanced workshops in the US and abroad. Dr. Joe is a faculty member at the International Quantum University for Integrative Medicine in Honolulu; the Omega Institute for Holistic Studies in Rhinebeck, New York; and Kripalu Center for Yoga and Health in Stockbridge, Massachusetts.

www.drjoedispenza.com

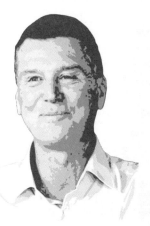

Mark D. Emerson, DC, CCSP
Author, Speaker, Lifestyle Medicine Expert

Dr. Mark Emerson specializes in nutrition-based lifestyle medicine and natural treatment methods for patients of all ages. Dr. Emerson has been a health and wellness consultant to players and personnel of the NFL, PGA Tour, USA Track and Field, and NCAA. Additionally, he provides private physician services to entertainment celebrities and Fortune 500 CEOs. As a Continuing Medical Education Provider (CME), Dr. Emerson has taught thousands of doctors and other allied healthcare providers evidence-based clinical nutrition protocols and blood lab interpretation to aid in the prevention and reversal of chronic progressive diseases such as cardiovascular disease and diabetes, as well as inflammatory and metabolic disorders.

www.docemerson.com

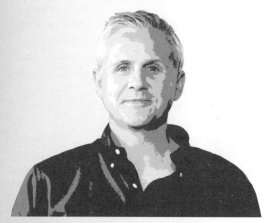

David R. Hamilton, PhD
Organic Chemist, Author

Dr. David Hamilton has a PhD in organic chemistry and spent four years in the pharmaceutical industry, developing drugs for cardiovascular disease and cancer. Inspired by the placebo effect, he left the industry to write books and educate people on how they can harness their mind and emotions to improve their health. He has authored nine books, including the bestsellers *How Your Mind Can Heal Your Body*, *I Heart Me*, and *The Five Side Effects of Kindness*. He writes a regular blog on his website and occasional blogs for the *Huffington Post* (US version) and *Psychologies* Life Labs. In 2016, he was voted best writer by readers of *Kindred Spirit* magazine.

www.drdavidhamilton.com

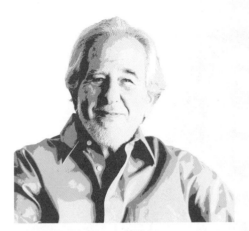

Bruce Lipton, PhD
Stem Cell Biologist, Author

Dr. Bruce Lipton is an internationally recognized leader in bridging science and spirit. A stem cell biologist, bestselling author of *The Biology of Belief,* and recipient of the 2009 Goi Peace Award, he has been a guest speaker on hundreds of television and radio shows, as well as keynote presenter for national and international conferences. His research at Stanford University's School of Medicine, between 1987 and 1992, revealed that the environment, operating through the membrane, controlled the behavior and physiology of the cell, turning genes on and off. His discoveries, which ran counter to the established scientific view that life is controlled by the genes, presaged one of today's most important fields of study, the science of epigenetics.

www.brucelipton.com

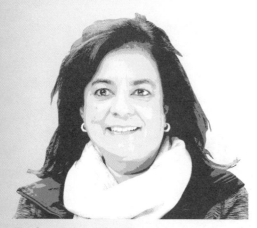

Anita Moorjani

Speaker, *New York Times* Bestselling Author

Anita Moorjani was born in Singapore of Indian parents and, at the age of two, moved to Hong Kong, where she has lived most of her life. She is multilingual and grew up speaking English, Cantonese, and an Indian dialect simultaneously; she later learned French at school. Anita had been working in the corporate world for many years before being diagnosed with cancer in April 2002. As a result of her near-death experience, Anita is often invited to speak at conferences and events around the globe. She is also a frequent guest at the University of Hong Kong's department of behavioral sciences, speaking on topics such as dealing with terminal illness, facing death, and the psychology of spiritual beliefs.

www.anitamoorjani.com

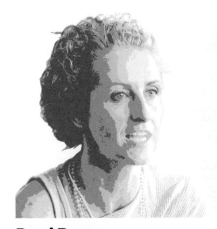

Patti Penn

Founder of Pause in Joy, Reiki Master, EFT Practitioner

Patti Penn is the founder of Pause in Joy, a spiritual-conscious community in Los Angeles with students worldwide. For more than a decade Patti channeled four workbooks with the Pause in Joy philosophy offering tools, energetic recalibration, and a reboot of re-trusting your intuition. Her emotional freedom technique (EFT) taps in, offering infinite possibilities, while out-creating old beliefs that were censoring choices. Her clients include veterans with PTSD, cancer patients who are or are not undergoing chemotherapy, and those dealing with anxiety, stress manifestations, trauma, anger, and fear.

www.pauseinjoy.com

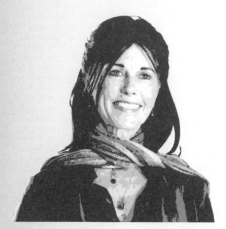

Dianne Porchia, MA, DMBM
Health and Wellness Coach, Mind/Body Medicine

Dianne Porchia's unique holistic somatic approach is the fast track to releasing past emotional hurt, trauma, and disempowering beliefs while effectively transforming an inner saboteur voice into an inner ally to support one's goals. Porchia works with many advanced-stage cancer patients and others going through stress-provoking challenges such as divorce, corporate burnout, death of a loved one, loss of job, and serious illness. Porchia's techniques include heart-centered communication skills, somatic dialogue, inner child healing work, sacred anger work, compassionate self-forgiveness, neurolinguistic programming (NLP), meditation, mindfulness, visualization, diaphragmatic breathing, and qigong. Porchia offers phone-FaceTime sessions, Life in Balance holistic wellness retreats, concierge services, and private retreats.

www.porchiaswish.com

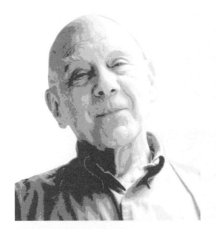

Bernie Siegel, MD
Author, Speaker

Dr. Bernie Siegel—who prefers to be called Bernie, not Dr. Siegel—was born in Brooklyn, New York. He attended Colgate University and Cornell University Medical College. He holds membership in two scholastic honor societies, Phi Beta Kappa and Alpha Omega Alpha, and graduated with honors. His surgical training took place at Yale New Haven Hospital, West Haven Veterans Hospital, and the Children's Hospital of Pittsburgh. He retired from practice as an assistant clinical professor of surgery at Yale (general and pediatric surgery) in 1989 to speak to patients and their caregivers. As a physician who has cared for and counseled innumerable people whose mortality has been threatened by an illness, Bernie embraces a philosophy of living and dying that stands at the forefront of the medical ethics and spiritual issues being grappled with today.

www.berniesiegelmd.com

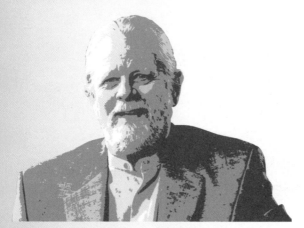

Jeffrey Thompson, DC, BFA
Neuroacoustic Wizard

Dr. Thompson is recognized as a worldwide expert in the field of acoustic pacing frequencies incorporated into musical soundtracks. A consummate musician and composer in his own right, he has established a method for using modulated sound pulses for changing states of consciousness, resulting in optimal mind-body healing. In the 1990s, Dr. Thompson's method of using sound to heal was chosen as one of the top alternative-healing modalities in the US. His work was funded through the Center for the Study of Complementary and Alternative Therapies (CSCAT). Dr. Thompson currently teaches at various institutions and through sponsored seminars, workshops, and certification courses.

www.scientificsounds.com

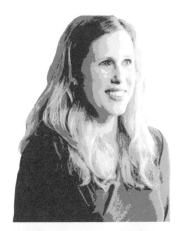

Kelly Turner, PhD
New York Times Bestselling Author

Dr. Kelly Turner is the *New York Times* bestselling author of *Radical Remission: Surviving Cancer against All Odds*, now published in twenty-two languages. Over the past decade, she has conducted research in ten different countries and analyzed more than 1,500 cases of radical remission. She holds a BA from Harvard University and a PhD from the University of California, Berkeley. Kelly has adapted her bestselling book into a fictional, feature-length screenplay titled *Open-Ended Ticket*. She is also working on a nine-part docuseries that will cover each of the nine key healing factors from her research, and feature many of the Radical Remission survivors from the book.

www.radicalremission.com

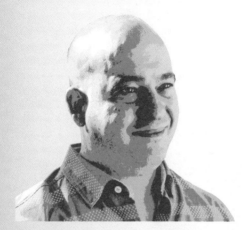

Darren Weissman, DC

Author, Founder of the LifeLine Center, Developer of The LifeLine Technique®

Dr. Darren Weissman is a chiropractic holistic physician, international speaker, and bestselling author. Dr. Weissman was named the Thought Leader for the United Breast Cancer Foundation and United Women's Health Alliance. He's been featured on Hay House Radio with his acclaimed radio show *The Heart of the Matter*, and has been featured in the films *E-Motion*, *Making Mankind*, *Beyond Belief*, and *The Truth*. Dr. Weissman developed The LifeLine Technique® in 2002. Since then, he established The LifeLine Center, offering a diverse array of individual care services and educational course programs devoted to personal development with a collective vision of creating world peace through inner peace. In addition, Dr. Weissman writes for magazines and blogs and maintains an international workshop and lecture schedule teaching The LifeLine Technique® via e-learning and live courses.

www.thelifelinecenter.com

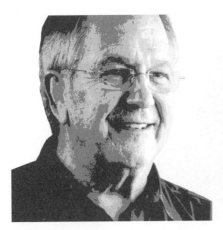

Rob Wergin
Divine Conduit

Rob Wergin is fully clairvoyant, clairsentient, and clairaudient. At a young age he was able to heal animals and communicate with spirits. These gifts were not understood, and he learned to ignore them. For more than thirty years he worked in corporate America as a highly successful CEO. Then one day he was hit by the ultimate "cosmic two-by-four," and in that time of deep despair, he asked what his life was for and . . . *he heard the answer*. Since then Rob has dedicated his life to being a vessel for divine light and love. He has helped tens of thousands of people of all ages and religions.

www.robwergin.com

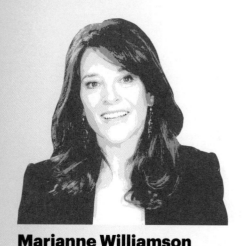

Marianne Williamson

Teacher, *New York Times* Bestselling Author

An internationally acclaimed lecturer, activist, and author of four #1 *New York Times* bestselling books, Marianne Williamson has been a well-known public voice for more than three decades. A quote from the megahit *A Return to Love*, beginning, "Our deepest fear is not that we are inadequate. Our deepest fear is that we are powerful beyond measure . . ." is considered an anthem for a contemporary generation of seekers. In 1989, she founded Project Angel Food, a meals-on-wheels program that serves homebound people with AIDS in the Los Angeles area. To date, Project Angel Food has served more than eleven million meals. Marianne also cofounded the Peace Alliance.

www.marianne.com

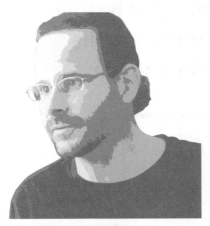

Anthony William

Medical Medium,
New York Times Bestselling Author

Anthony William was born with the unique ability to converse with a high-level spirit who provides him with extraordinarily accurate health information that's often far ahead of its time. When Anthony was four years old, he shocked his family by announcing at the dinner table that his symptom-free grandmother had lung cancer. Medical testing soon confirmed the diagnosis.

For more than twenty-five years, Anthony has devoted his life to helping people overcome and prevent illness—and discover the lives they were meant to live. He is the author of the *New York Times* bestseller *Medical Medium*.

www.medicalmedium.com

Now continue your healing journey and watch the award-winning film.

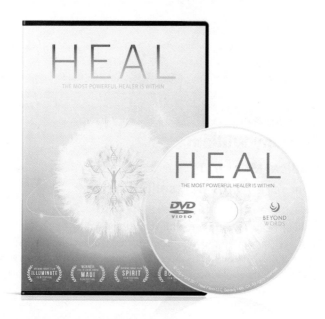

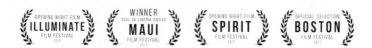

Order your DVD at beyondword.com/heal